BODY WITHOUT MYSTIQUE

PROMOTING HEALTH WITH THE WISDOM OF CHINESE MEDICINE

by Dr. Helen Hu

Copyright © 2011 by Helen H. Hu

All rights reserved.

No part of this book may be reproduced or stored in any form whatsoever without the prior written consent of the author.

Helen H. Hu

Printed in the United States of America

First Printing: February 2011

Body without Mystique 1

Table of Contents

Introduction 2
Chapter 1
    The History and Development of TCM Food Therapy 6
Chapter 2
    Basic Traditional Chinese Medicine Therapy 14
Chapter 3
    Basic Principles of Chinese Medicinal Nutrition 28
Chapter 4
    The Basic Concepts of Yao Shan and its Function 46
Chapter 5
    How to Apply Food Therapy According to Age 53
Chapter 6
    Food Therapy Modifications According to Seasonal Changes 87
Chapter 7
    Food Therapy According to Different Types of Body Constitutions 102
Chapter 8
    Food Therapy for Natural Detoxification 146

Introduction

"Return to nature," and "Humans and nature are one," represent the core philosophies of this book on the use of diet therapy to restore the body's energy and empower it for well-being and longevity. Humans exist between heaven and earth, a part of and supported by Mother Nature, which sustains life by providing many forms of healing energy on the planet. It depends on us to recognize and utilize it for the well-being of humanity. The universe (Tai: 太), which manifests the laws of nature and everything within it, consists of change from birth to death (Ji: 极), elucidating the laws of nature. No matter how everything changes, it must follow and stay within the laws of nature. This is the most essential part of the philosophy that Traditional Chinese Medicine and Daoism (Taoism) are based on.

The wellness and longevity of humans is part of the process of nature. In order to maximize physical and mental well-being, we need to change the way we treat ourselves, the way we think, and the way we treat the environment that we live in. At the same time, we have to recognize that no one lives forever; there is no "magic elixir" that enables us to become immortal. But we can age gracefully, in a natural and spiritual way. We must follow nature's law, that all life on the planet has its own life cycle. Mother Nature (the earth) provides nutritional energy (Qi) packed in "food" with healing powers. It depends on us to learn how to utilize it according to each individual's unique needs and capacities.

Our modern world, particularly in the past 50-70 years, has become more and more separate from nature, ignoring its laws. So, it is not surprising that many people have never had local, seasonal food and do not even know which fruits and vegetables belong to which season or region. We overeat and believe we can sustain ourselves only by consuming synthetic supplements; processed, packaged food; and artificially flavored and colored food and beverages that have lost their original energy (Qi) that Mother Earth provides. I call it "dead food"—food that is not only without any healing properties or Qi-supporting functions for our health, but is also harmful to our health.

Each of us, as a unique individual, as a part of nature, must follow nature's laws to empower our body and restore it to its maximum capacity. As we come to understand that Mother Earth provides herbs, plants, seeds, and nuts of all kinds, we will understand that to reach a maximum life span means knowing how to choose the right kinds of food to fit one's own natural body, empowering it for healing.

One might ask, what do you mean "empower" one's body for healing? As one of millions of forms of life on the earth, and like any other life form on the planet, humans possess the same self-healing power (which includes Essence, Qi, and Spirit) that Mother Earth provides for all of nature: the "energy" (Qi) that is packed in the form of herbs, water, soil, insects, and animals. It is left to us to know how to choose what we need. Empowering the body for healing is not simply adding a supplement to the body. Empowering the body means taking measures to restore and balance what the body already possesses—its natural healing capacity. (We must learn that, in certain circumstances, long-term use of supplements will, in fact, weaken or shut down the body's healing and adapting abilities.)

There is a saying in Chinese that "hundreds of illnesses enter via the mouth." This means that one way to promote well-being and longevity is through attention to the diet. Following a diet for longevity forms the theoretical basis of Chinese medicine. This entails the constant balancing of diet according to the body's constitution and ensuing physical changes, paying attention to what should be eaten and what should be avoided, and adjusting the intake amount of food in order to maintain health and promote longevity.

Whole food is the basic element needed for the survival of humans and all living things on earth. However, in our modern society, and especially in the West, we are only interested in the vitamins, fats, calories, and fiber content in our food, labeling food products with lists of these ingredients and creating a gigantic commercial market for vitamin and food supplements. But does this mean we are nourished by vitamins and supplements alone? Can we explain all the properties of foods solely by their vitamin content? Or is there something more to food that we don't understand? Obviously there is more to food than this, but what?

The theory of Traditional Chinese Medicine (TCM) is that the most vital components for life are Jing (physical body), Qi (energy), and Shen (spirit), the so-called "Three Treasures." A good diet not only nourishes our physical body and our organs, giving us vital energy, but it also nourishes our spirit. When Chinese medicine speaks of organs, it refers more to the energetic function of each organ than to anatomy only, as in Western medicine. If a person has weakness in a certain organ and an imbalance between organs, as part of the treatment, the diet can be modified to reestablish balance and strength.

Food has different tastes, which can be classified as sour, bitter, sweet, pungent, salty, and bland. Each taste corresponds to the promotion and nourishment of a particular organ function. For example, sour foods and herbs tend to correspond to the liver, bitter foods to the heart, pungent to the lungs, sweet to the spleen, and salt to the kidneys. As with different tastes, food also has different colors, each with corresponding tendencies to nourish different organs. For example, black-colored foods tend to nourish the kidneys, yellow foods tend to nourish the spleen, red foods correspond to the heart, green foods to the liver, and white foods to the lungs. In fact, Chinese medicine teaches that the kidneys are related to well-being, longevity, hair, bones, marrow, and hearing. So in order to nourish kidney function and promote well-being and longevity, it is beneficial to eat more black-colored foods, such as black beans, black sesame seeds, black rice, and other dark-colored foods. Modern-day research studies have shown that many black-colored foods promote health and prevent many diseases.

One's diet can also promote longevity by increasing immunity, preventing disease, helping to eliminate acute illness, and aiding in recovery from chronic disease. For example, eating animal liver prevents night blindness; seaweed provides iodine; fresh green onions and ginger prevent the common cold; and mung bean soup prevents summer heat stroke, as well as protects against pollutants.

In ancient times, people lived closer to nature in more integrated communities. Over thousands of years, through observation and by surviving many diseases and natural disasters, they discovered how various foods promote longevity and well-being. Many of these longevity-promoting foods and herbs have been recorded in the history of Chinese medicine, including sesame seeds (especially black sesame seeds), mulberries, walnuts, wild yams, wolfberries (goji berries), and yogurt, to name a few.

We are all familiar with the story of the father who teaches his son the skill of how to catch fish in order to empower him with a life skill, rather than just supplying him with fish to eat, making him dependent and incompetent his whole life. Learning how to utilize the natural substances provided by Mother Nature to empower the body for well-being and to promote longevity is an essential life skill for us all.

Chapter 1
The History and Development of TCM Food Therapy

Throughout all of human history, one of the most important turning points for human civilization was the introduction of fire.

The discovery of fire and its utilization to cook food for consumption was a milestone of human civilization. Cooked food not only made it easy for the body to break down or digest food for more efficient absorption, but more importantly, it eliminated a variety of infectious diseases and parasites. People also learned to use fire to ward off the cold of the winter months, as well as to treat cold-related diseases. There is no precise answer to when Traditional Chinese Medicine (TCM) began to develop, but it is believed that about 2200 BC, the Chinese people started using the earliest forms of herbs, acupuncture (with stone needles), and moxibustion, which involves burning herbs, most commonly mugwort, to warm up certain areas of the body for treating illness. They also used other modalities, such as hot stones to warm themselves and to ease pain. They understood that certain foods could relieve illness, while others were the cause of illness or were poisonous.

Around 1700 to 1100 BC, during the Shang dynasty, it is believed that one of China's earliest ancestors, Fu Xi, lived along the Yellow River of China. (According to legendary stories and mythology, Fu Xi is the ancestor of all Chinese people). By inscribing the oracle bones of buffalo and tortoise shells, he described a primitive principle of medicine, including methods for using wine and hot water as medicine, as well as the use of needles and bronze knives as surgical instruments. At that time, the Shang people believed that there was a relationship between humans, the heavens, and the earth. Their concept of the universe explained the laws of nature, which applied to humans and every other living thing on earth. According to this view, the five human internal organs correspond to the five elements: wood, fire, water, earth, and metal. Up until today, classic TCM teachings are still strongly based on this principal concept.

Inner Classic (*Nei Jing*), the only one of the earliest complete TCM books remaining today, was written by several authors from 300-100 BC (Chinese history indicates that many Chinese medicine books existed earlier that were more complete than *Inner Classic*, but none remain today). *Inner Classic* includes 18 chapters and 162 lessons. It describes how the basic laws of nature, the five elements, and yin and yang theory explain many aspects of human beings, such as physiology, pathology, diagnosis, treatment, and prevention of diseases. Two chapters specifically refer to Yang Sheng, the practice of nourishing life or longevity. Many sources record that the book was given to the Yellow Emperor (Hang Di) between 2698-2589 BC, and the Yellow Emperor read it and asked many questions to the superior Doctor Bian Que. One chapter of the *Inner Classic*, entitled "*Su Wen*" ("The Simple Question"), recorded the Yellow Emperor's question with the answer from Dr. Bian Que. Up until today, *Inner Classic* is still the most fundamental book taught in TCM schools, regardless of the modern technology we have today or how modified the version of TCM being practiced and taught in the West today. Without knowledge of the basic, fundamental principles of TCM, this modified version of TCM is only causing harm. Chinese medicine as a system developed gradually, and continues developing today, long after the first book was completed thousands of years ago.

Until about 221 BC, with the application of metal utensils and more advanced farming and technology, the ruling class was focused on Yang Sheng, and the promotion of personal and environmental hygiene, by balancing the diet in order to prevent disease. In fact, the ruling class developed a policy that enforced maintaining a particular diet to promote health and prevent epidemic disease.

At the same time, the three main religions in China—Daoism, Buddhism, and Confucianism—had their own ways of promoting Yang Sheng, with Daoism especially having a great influence on the "promotion of longevity" aspect of Chinese medicine. To some extent, Daoism philosophy is hard for Westerners to comprehend, and even more so, to practice. Daoism taught that in order to become immortal (live longer), one should be in the state of no-desire, no-self, and no-motivation, returning to the true state of simplicity (*pu shi*: 朴实), like a newborn. It is believed that the young and newborn may look weak, but have the potential power of life within. By contrast, when one matures and becomes stronger, it is a sign of aging.

The Daoists taught that to promote longevity, one should have a regular routine, maintain a disciplined diet, and lead a lifestyle that corresponds to the laws of nature, modified according to the four seasonal changes. In a word, regularity of lifestyle, discipline, a balanced diet, and attention to weather/seasonal changes ensure a long, healthy life. In contrast, irregularity of lifestyle, a diet without discipline, and ignoring weather, seasons, and environmental changes leads to exhausting the body and shortening life. However, one of most important essences of Yang Sheng from Daoism is the state of empty mind and inner peace.

Nan Bei Dynasty (265-581 AD): An organized medical system developed during this period, and the Emperor's Court of Officials was trained in a variety of medical specialties.

Tang Dynasty (618–907 AD): The collection and compilation began of the lost pieces/manuscripts of *Shang Han Lun*, one of the most well-known and studied books in TCM history, written by Dr. Zhang Zhong Jin. The development of the entire system of higher education (universities) for teaching and training TCM doctors began during this period.

This was the time of Dr. Sun Si Miao, the author of *Golden Chamber*, another one of the most widely studied books taught in Chinese medical schools. He lived to 134 years of age.

Song Dynasty (960-1279 AD): The completion and compilation of *Shang Han Lun* continued. There was continued development and refinement of TCM theory in internal medicine and pediatric (infant) medicine; more advances were made in the treatment of infectious disease; many groups of scholars of TCM arose.

Jin Dynasty (1115-1234 AD): Great leaps were made in the development of TCM and different theories. Four famous scholars emerged in this era of Chinese medicine: Dr. Liu Yuan Su, who developed and specialized in treatments with cold and cool herbal medicines; Dr. Zhang Cou Zheng, who developed and specialized in treatments with purgative herbal medicines; Dr. Li Dong Hen, who developed and specialized in treatments with warm, tonifying herbal medicines; and Dr. Zhu Dan Xi, who developed and specialized in treatments with tonifying, yin herbal medicines.

Ming Dynasty (1368-1644 AD): There was the continued refinement of TCM theory, with further exploration and creation of treatment strategies and new theories of diagnosis. A famous doctor of this era was Dr. Wang Kentang, who develop and specialized in pediatric medicine.

Qing Dynasty (1644-1912 AD): Early immunization in Chinese history started at 900 AD, but during the Qing dynasty, immunization became more developed and sophisticated. Immunization is applying the TCM principle, "Use toxin to conquer toxin." *Zhen Dou Ding Lun* ("Skin Lesion Diagnosis") by well-known Dr. Zhu Chuen Xia recorded that the immunizations against smallpox and measles were developed in southwest China, Sichuan Province, and Er Mei Mountain by Dr. Song Zhen Zhong (998-1022 AD). Local people called him a miracle doctor. He started to use the crest of smallpox lesions with many other detoxification herbs, ground together into a fine power, as a "vaccine." The instructions were to gently blow the fine powder into the nasal cavity to initiate immunity from the body against the smallpox outbreak. Dr. Song was invited to the palace to vaccinate Mr. Wang Su, the son of the Deputy of the Palace.

During the Qing dynasty in the early 18th century, a smallpox pandemic broke out over the entire world. In Europe alone, smallpox claimed over 150 million lives. Many of those who survived were left disfigured. The method of using live lesions to vaccinate against smallpox was started in Europe in 1796 by Dr. Edward Jenner.

Before the 18th century, TCM was a well-developed, sophisticated system of health care, clinical research, and education.

18th to 20th Centuries: Especially in the early 19th century, foreign powers such as the English, French, and Americans, who had previously negotiated unfair trade deals under the Qing dynasty, cheated China of her cultural heritage, aided by the corrupted, weakened Qing sovereignty. Westerners and Western cultural norms slowly pervaded the country, including the practice of Western medicine, which in large part was brought to China in the 1800s by Christian missionaries who set up hospitals and dispensed Western medicine. Chinese medicine suffered from both the Western invasion and from practices of some officials of the ruling party, the Kuomintang (KMT). According to KMT official Mr. Wang Da Xie, TCM was seen as a symbol of old, backward, unscientific, and fraudulent theories. He called for the abolishment of TCM, and limited or banned the advertisement and practice of Chinese medicine, prohibiting the teaching of Chinese medicine in medical schools and universities. Even today, there is resistance to or reluctance expressed by Westerners and scientists regarding the "legitimacy" of Traditional Chinese Medicine. Sadly, the primary motivation behind resistance to the practice of TCM in some

Western regions is economic in nature, with no regard to the health and wellness of the public.

1949-Present: After 1949, under the ruling of the Communist Party, the People's Republic of China abolished a thousand years of feudalism. One of the missions of the Chinese Communist Party was to provide free education and free medical care to the public. However, because of economic concerns, the government cannot afford the expensive development and research of new drugs like the West offers to the public. China already has a vast treasure of knowledge from the ancestors, with natural herbs that cost little compared with the cost of drugs. Therefore, it is very practical to promote TCM, vaccinate the masses freely, and educate the public via many channels on how to prevent diseases, such as practicing Tai Chi and Qigong, and broadcasting health tips to the public. Many Chinese know a slogan from Mao, the deceased head of the Communist Party: "TCM is our ancestors' treasure. We should maximize it and continue exploring and developing it."

In the medical schools and universities, TCM, Western medicine, and public health schools are on the same campuses, and the teaching of TCM and Western medicine is integrated. Doctors training in TCM have 40-45% of their coursework in Western medicine, and doctors training in Western medicine have 30-35% of their coursework in TCM. Doctors trained in Western medicine who treat patients with integrated medicine with an integrated approach fulfill the criteria to be promoted to doctor-in-charge, chief doctor, and/or professor. Additionally, further exploration, research, and development have occurred in herbal medicine, as well as development and research in acupuncture combined with technology.

The Chinese government has been promoting the teaching, research, and practice of TCM and continues to develop TCM to a new, advanced stage unparalleled in any era of Chinese history. TCM practitioners are not only exploring ways to treat certain diseases considered untreatable in the past, such as mute and deaf disorders, but also to face new challenges of treating diseases not seen before, such as AIDS and SARS (Severe Acute Respiratory Syndrome).

Today, research is carried out all over the world as scientists and physicists try to discover how and why acupuncture works, even though points and meridians do not exactly follow the nervous and vascular systems. We are still trying to explain how it works. In 1995, I happened to meet a Canadian physicist who was conducting meridian research at the California Institute for Human Science. The research project involved injecting an isotope at a point of the lung meridian at the tip of the thumb, and then trace it. Surprisingly, they discovered that the isotope injected at the tip of the thumb followed a path all the way to the lung. The pathway exactly followed the lung meridian as depicted on the Chinese acupuncture meridian map, but there is no nerve or blood vessel that follows the same path.

In the past two or three decades, a lot of TCM clinical research has been conducted in universities in many Western countries. I am not surprised that most of the research results are not impressive, or indicate that TCM does not work as people claim. The reason is that most of the research scientists do not understand that TCM works with the Qi (life force or energy), the body energy, as the basic element, and therefore its diagnoses and treatment principles revolve around the Qi, which is not tangible, not measurable, and not visible in a cadaver. One clinical symptom can be traced by many patterns of imbalance of organ and meridian systems. The treatment principle, therefore, is to balance the body accordingly in order to resolve the symptoms. In a word, a disease identified by one name in Western medicine can have many treatment options depending on TCM pattern differentiation on the diseases. However, on the opposite end, Western medicine is based on anatomy, using tangible evidence for its diagnosis and implementing treatment based on this evidence. Most of the mistakes made in such research projects result from using Western medicine research criteria to conduct TCM clinical trials, much like trying to use one key to open a different lock. This kind of "research," conducted by using anatomical, evidence-based research methods to measure energy- or Qi-based medicine, can only come to one conclusion: only biomedicine works. But recently, some researchers have started to recognize this and are trying to find a suitable method to conduct Qi-based clinical research.

Chapter 2
Basic Traditional Chinese Medicine Therapy

My goal in this book is not to teach Traditional Chinese Medicine. However, since we are going to talk about nutrition and its healing properties from the perspective of Chinese Medicine, it is necessary to understand some of the fundamental principles of TCM, so that you can make better dietary choices that suit you personally.

**The Basic Concept of Yin and Yang
and the Five Natural Elements, as Related to Humans**

In Chinese philosophy, the concept of yin and yang describes how polar or seemingly contrary forces are interconnected and interdependent in the natural world, and how they give rise to each other in turn. The concept lies at the heart of many branches of classical Chinese science and philosophy, as well as being a primary guideline and fundamental principle of Traditional Chinese Medicine. It is also a central principle of different forms of Chinese martial arts and exercise, such as Ba Gua Zhang (for telling and predicting the future), Tai Chi Chuan, Qigong, and I Ching divination. Many natural dualities—dark and light, female and male, low and high, cold and hot—are viewed in Chinese thought as manifestations of yin and yang respectively.

Yin and yang are complementary opposites within a greater whole. Everything has both yin and yang aspects that constantly interact; nothing ever existing in absolute stasis.

Daoism philosophy generally discounts good/bad distinctions as superficial labels, preferring to focus on the idea of balance. The idea that yin and yang have a moral dimension originated in the Confucian school, starting around the second century BC.

In Chinese Medicine, as in Daoism, it is believed that the heavens (sky, the space, or the universe), human beings, and the earth are one, and that this is the law of nature. The five elements—wood, fire, earth, metal, and water—follow the natural law of the five elements, which in turn explain each of our primary five organ functions, character, and position in relationship to the other organs. For example, water indicates the kidneys, which manifest, generate, and regulate water in the body. If water and fire (which indicates the heart) are not balanced, it means there is not enough water to control fire, and, according to natural law, more heat will be generated, and there will be too much heat in the body. If kidney energy is deficient, it cannot balance out the heat of the heart/fire, causing insomnia, anxiety, and uneasiness. Treatment of these symptoms should focus on nourishing water (the kidneys) and calming fire (the heart) in order to balance the two organs. As we can see, the treatment of insomnia in TCM does not directly target the brain cells in order to inhibit brain cell activity to induce sleep, but rather it aims to harmonize the organs.

Besides the principle of how the organs function, the essential core philosophy of Chinese medicine is yin and yang. The relationship between yin and yang is used to explain the principle of all change and movement in the universe, including the relationship of the body system to each of its organs; the body's immunity to pathogens; and the relationship of Qi (the yang aspect of energy) to Xue (the blood, a condensed form of Qi or yin material).

Deficiency and Excess – Cold and Hot

When TCM describes the concept of pathogens, it does not refer to bacterial and viral infection, but rather refers to anything that stresses the body, from emotional factors to environmental changes. In detail, pathogens include seven emotions and temperature states: wind, cold, heat (including summer heat and heat stroke), dampness, dryness, fire toxins, and internal stress from unrealistic desires and other mental activity (Shen/spirit status)

Diagnosis

In TCM, diagnosis is a very different process from that of Western bio-medicine today. In modern society, disease is diagnosed based on evidence produced by modern technology. In contrast, Traditional Chinese Medicine originated at least 4,000 years ago without any technology, using close observation of the body's signs and symptoms to evaluate how the mind and body perform in relation to an individual's energy cycle, dietary intake and output, emotions, and seasonal and weather changes. All the signs and symptoms the body manifests are due to internal organ imbalances. At this stage, it is a simple matter of making diet modification and lifestyle changes in order to balance the organs. Once organ balance is restored, all the signs and symptoms related to the imbalance are eliminated.

The progression of an imbalance in the body is a slow process, starting from a point of energy flow, and can have a variety of causes. At an early stage, however, no evidence will be detected by bio-medicine or today's modern technology. If the signs and symptoms are ignored just because no evidence is found by bio-medicine, then the disorders or imbalances of the body will gradually accumulate to the point of finally providing evidence that can be seen by today's technology. Once the body has built up the "evidence" which provides the sole source of diagnosis for bio-medicine, the body has already been ignored for a long period of time. At that point, an integrated medical approach can bring a maximized result by restoring the body's natural capacity and incurring less harm to the body. It is not hard to integrate all aspects of medicine together for the maximum well-being of humanity, but sadly, close-mindedness and, too often, *money* get in the way.

TCM rarely uses symptoms to name the diagnosis, but rather

the underlying organ disharmony. For this reason, it is called pattern diagnosis. When the body starts to show certain signs and symptoms that can be diagnosed by a TCM doctor, the pattern of each organ will be observed and determined, such as which organ is deficient and what is in excess: the heat, coldness, or dampness of each organ, and/or which kind of pathogen is blocking a meridian.

The concept of meridians is central to traditional Chinese medical techniques such as acupuncture, martial arts, Tai Chi, and Qigong. The theory of the channels or meridians is interrelated with the theory of the organs. The internal organs have never been regarded as independent anatomical entities. Rather, attention has centered upon the functional and pathological interrelationships between the channel network and the organs. So close is this identification that each of the twelve traditional primary channels bears the name of one or another of the vital organs.

The Organ Systems Relating to Health and Longevity

The Heart

In TCM, the functions of the heart are different from those of the anatomical heart as it is understood in Western medicine. The heart organ represents a group of physiological functions. In addition to regulating the cardiovascular system, it is responsible for maintaining the nervous system's functions.

"The heart rules the blood and blood vessels."

The heart is the functional unit for regulating blood flow. When the heart pumps, blood inside the blood vessels is transported around the entire body. The heart, blood, and blood vessels are united by their common activities. In TCM, this functional relationship is known as the "ruling" of the heart.

"Heart Qi" refers to the pumping action of the heart. If heart Qi is abundant and sufficient, and the heart pumps at a normal pace, transporting blood smoothly inside the blood vessels, then the pulse is regular and strong, and the facial complexion will be brilliant and vibrant. As a result, the body is able to obtain from the blood the nutrients needed to sustain life. On the other hand, if heart Qi is deficient, the blood cannot maintain an efficient flow in the blood vessels, and the pulse is weak. The individual looks pale, and the tongue also appears pale and white. Without healthy ruling of the heart, individuals will experience palpitations, chest discomfort, and pain.

"The heart rules the spirit."

In TCM, the heart stores the spirit. In general, "spirit" refers to an individual's vitality, which is reflected in the eyes, speech, reactions, and overall appearance. More specifically, the spirit refers to a person's mental, cognitive, and intellectual abilities. The heart takes charge of mental activities by mastering other organs and their physiological functions. If the ruling of spirit is well balanced, the individual will be wise and have a clear and sharp mind. If there is heart Qi and blood imbalanced within or disharmony with other organ, there might be signs of forgetfulness, poor self-esteem, and slow thought processes or reactions.

"Sweat is the fluid of the heart."

Sweat comes from body fluids, which are an essential and integral part of the blood. The blood is ruled by the heart and is the main fluid of this organ. Because sweat comes from the same origin as blood, in TCM, over-sweating is considered an exploitation of Qi and heart blood, leading to symptoms such as palpitations and dizziness. As a result, people who sweat abnormally usually have a heart deficiency. If such sweating is spontaneous, the disharmony belongs to a deficiency of heart yang energy. If it takes place at night, the disharmony belongs to a deficiency of heart yin energy.

According to TCM, the heart governs the blood and the vessels, ensuring the constant circulation of blood to all parts of the body, the same as in Western medicine. However, the heart also governs the spirit. In TCM, "spirit" means clarity of mind, strength and capacity of mental activity, inspiration, consciousness, self-awareness, and a certain emotional state. When heart Qi and blood are deficient, the clinical manifestations will include palpations, chest pain, emotional problems, manic depression, and sleeping disorder. Of course, in TCM, the heart function of governing spirit goes far beyond this, but this provides the general idea.

Even though Western medicine classifies mental consciousness and activity as functions of the brain, when a patient has heart disease and hypotension occurs, cerebral circulation is reduced, and mental consciousness or mental clarity declines. The intact functioning of the brain depends on the competent functioning of the heart, which provides sufficient oxygen to brain cells.

In TCM, certain foods nourish the heart, maintaining healthy heart functioning to ensure good circulation and a good spirit. This entails a variety of nutritional foods, principally consisting of plant proteins, while limiting sodium and animal fats.

Too much greasy food generates phlegm in the body (this can be mucus or fatty tissue). Phlegm can cause a great deal of damage in the body, including meridian blockage, which causes pain, or, if it is a blockage of the heart or blood vessel, the individual will suffer from heart or vascular disease. If phlegm causes mind or heart orifice blockage, it will manifest as a mental disorder. In Chinese medicine, it is believed that black soybeans, mushrooms, peanuts, ginger, onions, garlic, tea leaves, yogurt, kelp, hawthorn fruit, corn oil, and whole grains and vegetables address phlegm blockage.

An important factor is not only what we eat, but how we eat. Many longevity scholars advise against eating and drinking quickly, as well as overconsumption of food and drink. They counsel that one must drink when thirsty, taking in the substance slowly to avoid suddenly causing too much of a workload on the heart. It is also wise to avoid stimulating food and drink such as alcohol and coffee, and too much hot, spicy food, which overloads and disturbs the energy of the heart. Of course, moderate exercise, meditation, Tai Chi, and the enjoyment of soothing music and art all help to maintain a good spirit.

Liver

In Chinese medicine, the liver is the organ that stores and regulates the blood, is closely related to the menstrual cycle, and reaches orgasm during sexual activity. The liver is the master organ that ensures that the body's energy flows freely. If we are under a lot of stress, either externally or internally, the liver is the organ that will feel it first. As energy (Qi) stagnates in the liver, the liver loses its command of free-flowing Qi. The effects are mood swings, anger, frustration, repressed emotion, and feeling pain or pressure in the chest. Most women will experience PMS (premenstrual syndrome), and a high percentage of individuals will have digestive system disorders, such as being nervous eaters, having low or no appetite, heartburn, diarrhea, or constipation. All these symptoms are due to the inability of energy to flow freely, thus compromising the function of the digestive system. Whether the liver is healthy and balanced or not, it can be seen by the strength of the nails, the eyes, and the tendons.

It is said that the spirit of the liver—"the host of the ethereal soul"—is related to the capacity and ability to plan ahead, and a sense of direction in terms of what we are doing and where we are going with our lives.

Food that is rich in vitamins K, A, and C, such as fresh green vegetables and fruits, are the main factors in maintaining healthy liver function. Fish, eggs, animal liver, soy protein, and other easy-to-digest, high-quality proteins are healthy foods for the liver. Certain herbs can be taken as tea in order to clear toxins from the liver and prevent liver infection from contagious viruses. Avoiding the abuse of alcohol, toxic medication, and being constantly under stress are practical steps that can be taken in daily life to help maintain a healthy liver. Adding more fiber to the diet to ensure regular, daily bowel movements is another important key factor for a healthy liver. This allows the smooth movement of gastrointestinal fluids and the free secretion of all the digestive enzymes.

Healthy liver exercises include Tai Chi, Qigong, and slow, abdominal deep breathing while lying on the right side of the body.

The Spleen and Stomach

In Western physiology, the spleen is a large, vascular, lymphatic organ. It acts as a reservoir and filters the blood. It also plays a role in making blood early on in life. In TCM, the spleen does not perform these functions. Rather, it assists with digestion, blood coagulation, and fluid metabolism in the body.

"The spleen rules transformation and transportation."

Since the spleen is the primary organ responsible for digestion, its main function is to transform food into its essence, which is subsequently transformed into Qi and blood. Once the ingested food and liquids get into the body, the spleen extracts a pure nutritive essence from them. This essence is used for the production of Qi, blood, and fluids, which the spleen then transports throughout the body. Liquids extracted as pure nutritive essence are sent upward to the lungs for dissemination and redistribution. Some liquids, however, will descend to the kidneys and the bladder to be excreted as urine. Thus, the most important function of spleen is to transform the food we eat into Qi.

If the transformation and transportation functions of the spleen are harmonious, there will be abundant nutritive essence for Qi and blood, but if the spleen is in disharmony, its digestive powers will be affected. As a result, abdominal distention, pain, loose stools, and/or diarrhea and malaise occur.

"The spleen rules ascending pure essence."

After transforming food into nutritive essence, the spleen sends it upward to the heart and lungs, where it is transformed into Qi and blood for nourishment of the whole body. Food not transformed into nutritive essence becomes an impure substance. While the spleen ascends pure essence, the stomach, the spleen's corresponding exterior organ, will descend the impure substances inside the digestive tract. By ascending the pure nutritive essence and descending the impure substances, a balance in the digestive system is created.

"The spleen governs the blood."

Not only does the spleen transform food essence, it also governs the movement of the blood by keeping it flowing in its proper pathways inside the blood vessels. When spleen Qi is sufficient, there is adequate production of Qi and blood, and blood remains inside the blood vessels. If the spleen's functions are in disharmony, the blood escapes from its normal pathways, leading to symptoms such as bloody vomit, blood in the stool, blood under the skin, blood in the urine, or menorrhagia (excessive menstrual bleeding).

"The spleen rules the muscles and flesh. It opens into the mouth, and its vitality is manifested in the lips."

In TCM, the movements of the muscles and the four limbs depend on the power of the spleen. When spleen Qi is sufficient, the limbs and muscles are healthy and strong because they are nourished by the blood with abundant Qi. However, if spleen Qi is deficient, the muscles become weak, and an individual may feel tired and have general malaise.

The lips and mouth are also affected by the spleen's health. If spleen function is harmonious, the mouth can distinguish the five tastes—sweet, salty, sour, bitter, and pungent or spicy—and the lips appear red and moist. If the spleen is weak, the mouth cannot distinguish the different tastes, and the lips will be pale.

The Lungs

In Western physiology, the lungs are responsible for air exchange. In addition to performing respiration, in TCM, the lungs also regulate fluid metabolism and control blood vessels, the autonomic nervous system, and the immune system (defensive system).

"The lungs rule Qi and administer respiration."

The lungs are where Qi exchange and regulation occurs. During inhalation, the lungs take in natural air Qi (one type of Qi referring to the atmospheric air), propelling it downward, where it meets other types of Qi. The different types of Qi combine to produce normal Qi (Qi present in the body). During exhalation, the lung expels the "impure" air that is not useful to the body. If the lungs are healthy, Qi will enter the body smoothly, and respiration will be even and regular. If there is lung disharmony, respiration is weakened, and normal Qi production is affected, leading to Qi deficiency.

"The lungs direct movement in a disseminating, descending, and liquefying manner."

The lungs disseminate substances in an ascending and outward direction. For example, impure air is expelled in this manner, and body fluids and food nutritive essence are directed toward the skin and hair. By regulating sweat secretion, the lungs disseminate protective Qi (responsible mainly for immunity) to the skin and the pores.

The lungs also demonstrate descending and liquefying properties. They take in natural air Qi during respiration and liquefy the fluids in the airways. The lungs then descend these substances downward, along with food essence transformed by the spleen. The descending function is necessary to maintain a normal respiratory tract.

The disseminating, descending, and liquefying properties of the lungs are essential for good health. If disharmony occurs, individuals may suffer from coughing, wheezing, chest discomfort, abnormal sweating, or congestion from phlegm.

"The lungs move and adjust the water channels."

The lungs are responsible for the transformation and movement of water in the body. They move water in the same directions as Qi. The lungs' disseminating properties enable water vapor to ascend and scatter to the skin pores. This is the process of normal sweating. The lungs also liquefy and cause water vapor to descend to the kidneys, where the liquefied waste is excreted as urine.

"The lungs collect blood vessels and rule Qi regulation."

As mentioned before, the lungs rule Qi. By regulating Qi movement that is necessary for blood circulation to occur, the lungs intercept all blood and blood vessels. After Qi exchange occurs during breathing, the Qi moves the blood throughout the body. Qi movement also regulates the distribution of body fluids. Since Qi is essential for all physiological functions in the body, the lungs' ability to rule and regulate Qi is an important function.

"The lungs open into the nose, and their vitality is manifested in the body's hair. The lungs also connect to the throat."

The skin and body hair share a close relationship with the lungs. Together with the sweat glands, they are often referred to as the "exterior" of the body in TCM. The lungs are the interior organs that rule this exterior. By controlling the skin, sweat glands, and body hair, the lungs regulate the sweating process. In addition, they maintain healthy movement and dissemination of protective Qi over the skin. Protective Qi is important for guarding the body against "illness evils" (factors causing illness, including wind, fire, dampness, dryness, cold, and summer heat). If these particular lung functions are weakened, too much spontaneous sweating occurs, and the protective Qi will become weak as well. As a result, the body will have lower resistance to illness and may easily get colds, influenza, or other respiratory problems.

The nose is considered the opening of the lungs and the exit for Qi in the body. If lung dysfunction occurs, the nose is affected. For example, disordered flow of lung Qi leads to a watery nasal discharge, congestion, a loss of sense of smell, and sneezing. The throat and vocal cords are also connected to the lungs. Sometimes lung deficiency produces a coarse or low voice.

The Kidneys

In Western physiology, the kidneys are vital excretory organs whose main function is to create urine to help the body get rid of toxins and unwanted water. TCM practitioners view the kidneys as very important organs that not only regulate the urinary system, but also exercise control over the reproductive, endocrine, and nervous systems.

"The kidneys store Jing."

In TCM, "Jing" (精) is the Chinese word for "essence," an essential substance closely associated with life. Jing is stored in the kidneys and is the densest physical matter within the body needed for reproduction, growth, development, and maturation. The kidneys are the organs responsible for human development, because they store Jing (essence). For example, conception is possible by the power of Jing; growth to maturity is the blossoming of Jing; and aging reflects the weakening of Jing. As time passes, Jing decreases and causes both vitality and kidney Qi to decline. This decline is the normal aging process.

"The kidneys rule water."

The kidneys rule water by regulating its distribution and excretion, traditionally described as the vaporizing power of the kidneys. The kidneys can differentiate between clean water that is recycled and used by the body, and turbid water that is turned into urine. The separation of these two is the vaporization process.

The kidneys play an important role in water movement and balance of the whole body. Fluids and food are received by the stomach, where separation begins. The unusable portions of foods and fluids are sent to the intestines as waste, where pure fluids (mainly water) are extracted from them. The pure fluids go to the spleen, which then sends them in a vaporized state upward to the lungs. The lungs circulate and disseminate the clear part of the fluids throughout the body. Whatever has become impure through use is liquefied by the lungs and sent downward to the kidneys. In the kidneys, the impure fluids are further separated into "clean" and "turbid" parts. The clean part is vaporized into a mist and sent upward to the lungs, where it rejoins the cycle. The final impure portion goes to the bladder, where it is stored and finally excreted as urine.

"The kidneys rule the grasping of Qi."

Although respiratory functions mainly depend on the lungs, deep and normal breathing is controlled by the "grasping" function of the kidneys. By grasping Qi, the kidneys enable the "natural air Qi" of the lungs to penetrate deeply during the inhalation process. If there is kidney disharmony, respiratory problems such as shallow breathing or wheezing upon exertion can occur. Some types of asthma are related to disorder grasping of Qi by the kidneys.

"The kidneys rule the bones and produce bone marrow."

Stored in the kidneys, Jing is the substance responsible for producing bone marrow, which in turn creates and supports bone growth. Therefore, bone development and repair depends on the nourishment of kidney Jing. Deficiency of Jing in children can lead to soft bones or incomplete closure of the skull bones. Teeth are made up of bone, so dental problems can also indicate a kidney deficiency.

"The kidneys manifest in the head hair."

Head hair depends on blood for its nourishment. The kidneys play a role in transforming stored Jing into blood. If Jing and blood are abundant, the hair will appear bright, shiny, and healthy. On the other hand, hair loss or other hair disorders can indicate a kidney deficiency or blood deficiency.

"The kidneys open into the ears and genital organs."

Good hearing comes with abundant kidney Jing, while a deficiency causes hearing problems, such as deafness or ringing in the ears (tinnitus). Genital and urinary tract disorders, such as urinary frequency or dripping urine (incontinence), are also signs of kidney disharmony.

Chapter 3
Basic Principles of Chinese Medicinal Nutrition

If you were to visit China and discuss food and nutrition with the people there, you would encounter a totally different perspective from that in the West. Rather than being interested in the vitamin or fiber content, or the number of calories in their food choices, they would want to know the taste, smell, and appearance of the food. They would ask, "What is the property (the proper function) of the food?" The "property" indicates how the food will interact with the body therapeutically, a concept that goes beyond that of nutritional value. The proper function of food is based upon the TCM classification of plants and other categories of food by five tastes, four Qi (temperatures), the energy direction of the food, and the main organ that the food targets. These characteristic properties provide information about the food's nutritional and medicinal value and function, and form the basis of traditional Chinese medicinal nutrition.

An ancient Chinese saying is, "Medicinal herbs and food come from the same source."

There are many herbs in TCM herbal formulas with which we are familiar, since we use them as spices, or simply as food, in our daily cooking. Some examples are ginger, clove, cinnamon, cumin, mint, garlic, green onion, and so on. Of course, there are many herbs we do not use on a daily basis that can be added into the diet to address specific medical conditions or to promote longevity. For example, black beans and dark grains nourish the kidneys energetically and promote longevity. Pears moisten the throat and benefit the lungs. Sweet rice nourishes the spleen. Bitter melon clears toxins from the body, as does green tea.

Growing up in China, I remember the hot and humid summers every year. In order to prevent summer heat stroke, Chinese families knew to make mung bean soup with a little bit of crystal rock sugar. During the winter, when children were susceptible to catching colds or the flu, to prevent an epidemic, the schools would make herb broths for them to drink, with green onion root, ginger root, Napa cabbage root, and some other herbs. It was mandatory for all students to drink the herb broth during recess.

It can be argued that with air conditioning to keep us cool in summer and vaccines to prevent flu and epidemics in winter, there is no need for the traditional practice of drinking herbal teas and broths. Of course, personal preference and choice should be respected, but with the prevalence of summer colds and respiratory problems in the modern world, it is important to recognize the effects that air conditioning can have on the body. In the late spring and early summer, the body's biological clock triggers increased consumption of the body's stored energy. During the summer, the body should be naturally perspiring in order to cleanse and discharge toxins. At the same time, the tendency to drink more cold fluids and eat more fresh fruits in the summer also cleanses and detoxifies the body. Air conditioning—especially making the room too cold compared to outside temperatures—will cause the body to work against its natural rhythm of adjustment, through which it achieves homeostasis in response to seasonal change.

Drinking mung bean soup to clear summer heat is just one aspect of the beauty of the mung bean. Not only does it clear heat, but it also clears toxins that our bodies absorb from environmental pollution and contamination, particularly pesticides. Additionally, as documented in Dr. Steven Pratt's *SuperFoods Rx,* mung beans, which are high in protein, also have the lowest ratio of calories to protein of the legumes and beans.

The important point I wish to make here refers to the TCM principle mentioned earlier: *Return to nature*. This means understanding and making use of the resources nature provides us with. It means learning how to integrate this knowledge into our daily lives through food choices and diets that heal in a natural way. Finally, it means understanding how to live healthier, longer lives.

The Basic Concepts of TCM Nutrition, or the Chinese Medicinal Diet

If I were to ask what drives your decision to buy particular fruits or vegetables when you go to the farmer's market or the grocery store, you might answer that you look for food that appears fresh, ripe, and in season; food that has a nice color or aroma or that tastes good, or maybe food that you know how to cook. Most likely, the last thing on your mind is, "I'm going to buy something with a full load of vitamins and minerals today." Why?

Food in today's world is valued according to its micro-content: its vitamins, antioxidant properties, minerals, and so on. Food is broken down into molecular units. Even so, in the thousands of years of human life on this Earth, most of us still relate to our food in a direct, sensual way—by its smell, taste, and texture. By doing so, we are able to relate directly to our food as something from nature, with natural origins. So which way is the "right way" to relate to food? A combination of both!

1) TCM views food as wholesome—as macro, energetic, original, and natural.

In TCM, the word "nutrient" or "nutritious" means holistic, which means something simple and natural that provides sustenance and well-being. It derives from the basic principle of the sky, nature, and human beings all being part of one universe. Just as all living things, all of life, must follow nature's cycle of birth, growth, aging, and death, so too the human body must follow this law of nature.

Macro: The Chinese herbal system uses and classifies plants as a whole, valuing all their therapeutic, supporting, and healing properties according to color and taste. Different parts of the plant carry different properties, such as the seed, root, leaf, and stem. The roots carry the supporting energy of the plant, like the ginseng root. The seeds, including beans, nuts, and grains, carry the potential energy for growth and nourishment. The blossom carries the energy upward, as in the chrysanthemum flower that clears heat from the face. The principle is: *One plant, one universe.*

Energetic: Different foods carry different energies that provide nutrition to, and affect the function of, different body organs and systems. The energy affecting the organ's function can be descending or ascending.

Original and Natural: This refers to recognizing food's distinct taste, color, smell, and distinct biological clock for maturation according to the season and geography in which it thrives. Plants, as a form of life on earth, follow the same natural law of birth and sprouting, growth and maturation, aging and death. Each cycle of the plant's life has different therapeutic and nutritional properties.

Many years ago, I visited a temple in northern China with an herbalist. While we walked along a deep path inside the garden with ginkgo trees on both sides, he pointed to ginkgo leaves that had fallen to the ground with a slightly yellowish color. He asked me, "What is the difference between the ginkgo leaves that are still on the tree and the ones that fall to the ground?" I never knew there was a difference! He told me that the ones still on the tree were not yet mature and still contained some poisons, but the ones that had fallen to the ground were without poisons and were appropriate for medicinal use. So we can only use ginkgo leaves at the end of their life cycle for therapeutic purposes.

Here is another example. Some of us know honeysuckle flower (*jin yin hua*), one of the most potent Chinese herbs used for eliminating heat and accumulated toxins from the human body, for conditions such as sore throat, acute bronchitis, and bacterial infection (lesion with pus – heat toxin lesion). The potent ingredient in the flower is at its most concentrated before the flower fully blooms; it loses its potent therapeutic function after the flower blooms. These two examples demonstrate how the different stages of a plant's life cycle carry different therapeutic properties and strengths of those properties.

Take a food that we are very familiar with, such as the tomato. If we pick a tomato too early, while it is still green, and do not allow the fruit to finish its natural biological life cycle, the fruit has to stop photosynthesizing and extracting nutrition from the earth. The tomato not only has no taste but no "fully packed" nutrients.

Several years ago, I visited Pele Mountain Organic Coffee Ranch in Kona, Hawaii. The owner taught me a good lesson during a tour of her farm. As we walked among the coffee trees, I saw all the coffee berries hanging on the branches like bundles of grapes. There were red- and green-colored berries, and berries that were in between, with both colors mixed. She picked a red berry from a branch and asked me to taste it. There was a little sweet-tasting sap on the peel of the coffee bean. She told me that when the berry on the tree becomes red, it is ready to be picked. The bean inside the shell will slowly absorb the sweet sap in the peel, so they let the red berry dry naturally without peeling it until a customer puts in an order. This allows the coffee bean to fully mature with its naturally sweet, soft taste, without the acidity that causes a caffeine surge when the coffee is ingested. Green, unripened coffee beans will taste strongly acidic and ensure a harsh caffeine reaction as a result.

However, picking only red coffee berries is a very slow process requiring intense labor. The farm owner explained that the coffee sold in big chain coffee stores and organic individual coffee shops in Kona come from the same kinds of coffee trees. The difference is whether the growers pick only the mature red berries or all the berries from the branch, including the green ones. I never forgot this lesson that taught me to recognize what a difference it makes when we ignore the natural life cycles of plants.

Geography: Originally, specific plants grew in specific geographical areas. When grown in a different climate or environment from that of their origin, these same plants carry different properties. For example, Siberian ginseng carries a very warm property, because it has to survive in a very cold climate in the wild. When our body suffers a cold and deficiency type of disorder, we can take Siberian ginseng to counter it. On the other hand, a mint plan with a cold property mostly grows in warm weather to balance its environment. If we plant Siberian ginseng in warm weather, it will change its property or might not grow at all. When we plant the same herb in a different geographical environment, the property of the herb will be changed to a certain degree because the plant has to change or adjust its inner environment or its biochemical makeup to survive this changed environment. The changed inner environment and biochemical makeup will result in a changed therapeutic property, in terms of Chinese herbology.

One example of a plant in Chinese Medicine, *chuan bei mu* (*Fritillaria cirrhosa bulbus*), grows in the Sichuan providence, a hot weather environment, which gives the plant *Fritillaria cirrhosa bulbus* a cool property to suit its environment. The herb is used for symptoms of heat and chronic coughing with dry or yellow mucus, with the property of moisturizing and nourishing the lungs. Meanwhile, the same plant, but grown in Zhe Jiang province, called *zhe bei mu* (*Bulbus fritillariae thunbergii*), is used for symptoms of heat and acute coughing and lung disorders.

Sometimes I am asked for my definition of organic food. I had always been happy to find that many people were interested in organic food, and I thought that my patients, as well as the audience members at my lectures, had the same idea of what this meant that I did. But after asking about their definition of organic food, I discovered that we had slightly different concepts about what constitutes organic food.

Most people believe that organic food is food that is free of pesticides, chemicals, and synthetic fertilizers—and they are absolutely right about that. However, one of the most important elements of organic food is that the plants are allowed to grow in their own original geographical area and according to their proper season until they are fully mature. This is nature's law, that each plant has its own biological clock, and nature must be allowed to take its own course.

In Traditional Chinese Medicine, it is believed that every living thing—including all the plants and animals on this planet—has its own natural course (or biological clock) that no one should change. This is the law of Mother Nature, and should anyone try to change it, they will be punished in one way or another as a consequence. All plants on this earth naturally grow in certain geographical areas, with a particular temperature, season, and soil type specific to it. Plants must be allowed to grow to full term so that they have enough time to collect and transform Qi (energy) from the sun (collecting and transforming light and oxygen) and the earth (collecting and transforming water and nutrients), forming nutrients that become the plant's own. Then the plant—fruit, seeds, and vegetables—can be harvested for human consumption, fully mature and rich with nutrients. This is what I call organic food, rather than food that may be chemical-free but has been prevented from growing to its full term in its original environment.

Where I grew up in northern China, every Chinese family made dumplings on New Year's Eve. The best dumpling recipe was made with a combination of lamb and Chinese chives. However, the fresh, green color of Chinese chives didn't grow in the wintertime for lack of sunlight. The only chives we could get during the winter were a pale yellow color and were grown in greenhouses. When the plant does not have its original, normal, vibrant color, it indicates that the plant is malnourished and lacks nutrients due to not having been grown in its optimal, most suitable environment.

Certain foods must grow in certain areas. When plants are relocated to a different area, their nutrients may change, or their nutritional value may be reduced compared to plants grown in their original, natural geographical area. Growing up in northern China, I remember everyone knew that the best snowflake pear came from Zhao County. The snowflake pear is very sweet and juicy, each pear weighing almost a pound. When other counties grew the same pear, even in the same province, the pears were never as tasty as those from Zhao County.

Likewise, the tastiest imaginable peaches came from Shen County, in China's Hebei Province. These large peaches were provided exclusively to royal families for hundreds of years, growing only in a few villages in Shen County. The peaches were a milky white color, with a red tip at the bottom. They were very large in size, and very sweet and juicy. When I went back to visit China in the year 2000, I asked my uncle about the big peaches of Shen County. I was very sad to hear him say that, for some reason, the area that had grown these special peaches had shrunk every year, until about five years prior, around 1995, when there were no more peach trees in those villages. My uncle suggested that environmental changes and fertilizer usage may have been contributing factors in damaging the soil, causing the famous peaches of Shen County to become a thing of the past.

In Chinese medicine, plants are used for medicinal purposes, and when a Chinese herbalist prescribes an herb, he or she will indicate the providence of the herb specified in the formula. This is because of the importance of the geographical origin of plants and the understanding that the nutritional content and the properties, as well as the function of herbs and plants, can differ according to the province in which they have been grown.

So eat local food and support local farms for better health.

2) TCM nutrition and TCM food therapy arise from the explanation and classification of food and nutrition in Traditional Chinese Medicine.

The theoretical basis of traditional Chinese nutrition is identical to how our ancestors saw food: as part of nature. Two thousand years ago, the classic TCM text, *Inner Classic*, already indicated how the five flavors of food correspond to different organs. TCM doctors applied TCM theory to prescribe food therapies in order to tonify or sedate, balance the yin and yang of the body for disease prevention, and enhance body performance and well-being. TCM therapies were developed for the ruling classes in particular. However, throughout all of Chinese history, all religions, such as Daoism, Buddhism, and Confucianism, as well as practitioners of the martial arts, adapted and utilized TCM food therapy in their daily practices. They all developed different characteristic recipes for food therapy, such as Daoist longevity therapy and the special diets in Buddhism. (To this day, Daoists practice Qi and Daoist food therapy for longevity, and even immortality.)

3) Being part of nature, TCM food therapy follows the laws of nature.

TCM food therapy is tailored to the individual according to one's life stage (age), gender, physical condition (such as pregnancy or recovering from surgery or chemotherapy), individual constitution, and type and stage of disease.

4) Nutrition in TCM shares the TCM principle of having the capacity to balance the yin and yang of the body.

TCM food therapy and nutrition are part of the whole that is Traditional Chinese Medicine, which includes herbal therapy, acupuncture, moxibustion therapy, Qigong therapy, and Tui Na (acupressure massage) therapy. A doctor who practices TCM should apply all the TCM tools for healing.

TCM food therapy and nutrition recommends that:

- A person who has more fire toxin in the body should not eat spicy, pungent, or hot foods;
- A person who has too much phlegm (fat) in the body should avoid phlegm (fatty) foods;
- A person with skin allergies and asthma should avoid shrimp, shellfish, and crab; and
- A person with cold stomach disorder should try to avoid cold and raw foods.

5) The wisdom of thousands of years of TCM history asserts that: *Food and herbs are from the same source.*

This has two meanings. First, herbs, plants, fruits, and all foods have certain characteristics of taste, color, smell, and shape; and second, herbs and all foods are classified according to their properties (as discussed below) in order to identify their therapeutic functions according to TCM theory. TCM uses certain spices as herbs, including ginger, green onions, garlic, cinnamon bark, clove, and fennel seeds. It also uses fruit as herbs, including goji berries, mulberries, hawthorn fruit, dates, longan, and wild Chinese yam.

Traditional Chinese Medicine teaches that humans are in the middle of the universe, nourished by heaven and earth. Here, "heaven" means the natural universe, which surrounds humans with *da Qi* (big energy), which supports all life on earth. Another important concept is that natural plants (representing a particular life form on earth) have the capacity to transform energy from heaven (sunlight/unformed energy) and store it as plant pigment (formed energy). This is then utilized as a source of energy by other forms of life, including human, that consume the formed energy stored in the plants. This is why the outer skin, or peel, of plants and fruits has more nutrients than the inner part, since the outer part is exposed directly to the sun. We know that when we plant trees or grow vegetables or fruits with little or no exposure to sunlight, the color of the plant looks pale compared to plants grown with full sun exposure. The more sun exposure the plants have, the darker and healthier the color of the plants and the more nutrients stored in the plant through photosynthesis. In other words, the more heaven energy (sun energy) transformed by the plant or fruit, the more heaven energy stored within the plant.

That is why TCM teaches that black-colored fruit nourishes kidney energy, which is vital to our well-being, longevity, development, productivity, sexuality, bone structure, and central nervous system. These foods include blueberries, blackberries, black beans, black rice, black sesame seeds, dark grapes—and black ants! Recently, the magazine *Life Extension* featured an article about research indicating that blueberries can help prevent Alzheimer's disease. Here we see how modern research has begun to prove what TCM claimed thousands of years ago. Blueberries (dark-colored fruit) nourish the kidneys, which are related to the central nervous system and the aging and longevity process.

Function and Classification of Food in TCM:
The Four Qi, Five Tastes, Energy Direction, Meridians,
and Properties of Tonifying and Sedating

The Four Temperatures (Four Qi) of Food

Chinese medicine categorizes food and herbs into four Qi, or four characteristic temperatures: cool, cold, warm, and hot. There are also neutral foods. In reality, we generally use three categories: cold (including cool), hot (including warm), and neutral (or bland) food. The temperature (Qi) of most foods is neutral; a smaller number of foods are classified as hot, and even less common are foods classified as cold.

1) **Cold foods** clear heat from the body (or detoxify), nourishing bodily fluids and the yin aspect of the body. Some examples of this food category are bitter melon, dandelion, lotus root, water chestnuts, seaweed, kelp, tomatoes, persimmons, tangerine peel, watermelon, bananas, mulberries, cucumbers, and snails.

2) **Cool foods** (less cold than cold foods) include eggplants, turnips, bok choy, spinach, celery, millet, barley, tofu, mung beans, wheat, apples, pears, mangoes, loquat, duck eggs, and mushrooms.

3) **Hot foods**, in general, have the function of warming the body, expelling body coldness and cold-related pain, increasing circulation, opening meridian and sinus blockages, and promoting organ function and the yang aspect of the body. Some examples of hot foods are cayenne pepper, mustard, Sichuan peppers, and cinnamon.

4) **Warm foods** (less warm than hot foods) include a broader variety of foods, such as garlic, chives, ginger, liver, green onions, fennel, almonds, longan, peaches, cherries, walnuts, plums, chestnuts, chicken, shrimp, lamb, deer meat, and goose eggs.

5) **Neutral foods** (or bland foods) usually can be consumed cooked or cold. Many foods belong to this category, including onions, potatoes, sweet potatoes, carrots, green beans, Napa cabbage, black beans, red beans, soybeans, peanuts, black sesame seeds, grapes, black fungus mushroom, white fungus

mushroom, fish, pork, duck meat, chicken eggs, honey, organic beef, and milk.

The Five Flavors (Five Tastes) of Food

Chinese medicine classifies food into five flavors, each relating to the five organs (heart, liver, spleen, lung, and kidney). The five flavors of food include: *sour, bitter, sweet, pungent,* and *salty*. (*Bland* is an additional taste that is sometimes included on this list.) Besides the five flavors, there is another category called **fragrance**, which refers to the smell or aroma of the food. Each of the different flavors, or tastes, of food has a different function.

1) **Sour-tasting food** has a consolidating, stringent function that ensures there is no leakage in the body. Examples of leakages might be some patterns of diarrhea, urinary leakage, premature ejaculation, and sweating easily. Foods in this category include tomatoes, vinegar, papayas, hawthorn berries, pomegranates, grapes, citrus fruits, peaches, and pears.

2) **Bitter-tasting food** has the function of draining downward. If there is a toxin in the body that needs to be drained, certain bitter-tasting foods can help detoxify, and some foods in this category can help inhibit cancer cells and viruses. These include bitter melon, *Portulacae oleraceae* (*ma chi qian*), dandelion, *Lycium chinesea mill* (goji tender plant), bitter tea leaves, green tea, ginkgo seeds, apricot kernels, lily bulbs, kelp, and certain vinegars and wines.

3) **Sweet-tasting food** has the function of tonifying and supplementing. We all know that when we are feeling tired or fatigued, we crave food from the sweet category for instant energy, or tonifying energy. Most food falls into this category,

including tomatoes, onions, carrots, potatoes, pumpkin, cabbage, cucumbers, cinnamon, beans (legumes), fruit, grains, and most meats.

4) **Pungent food** has a dissipating, evaporating function. For example, after catching a cold, we have body aches, and we may begin to perspire as our body surface releases sweat. TCM calls it "expelling the pathogen through sweating." Then, if we drink hot soup with pungent herbs, such as ginger, green onions, and some pepper, it helps to open the sweat glands, facilitating the dispersion or evaporation of toxins through perspiration. After sweating, the body feels released. Many kitchen spices are included in this category of food, such as ginger, green onions, cilantro, mustard, horseradish, turnip seeds, garlic, chives, cinnamon, tangerine peel, and cayenne pepper.

5) **Salty-tasting food** has the function of softening nodules and hardness. The salt carries moisture into the hard mass, which is why Chinese herbalists always use plants from the sea, or other salty-tasting herbs, to treat masses in the body. These foods include sea salt, millet, rice, seaweed, kelp, seafood, pork, ham, and duck meat.

Classifying the Five Flavors and Colors of Food According to Meridians

TCM also classifies food according to which meridian the food belongs to. This is one of the very basic nutritional characteristics of TCM. Based on this theory, TCM doctors will advise what kinds of food the patient needs in his or her diet, according to the patient's condition.

- **Foods belonging to the heart meridian:** According to TCM theory, in most cases, *bitter-tasting* and *red-colored* foods belong to the heart meridian. Of the five elements, the heart element is fire (red color), and a bitter taste can drain fire down, balancing it. Therefore, following this principle, red-colored and bitter-tasting foods tend to correspond to the heart organ. These include cayenne pepper, red beans, and certain kinds of mushrooms, watermelon, sour dates, longan, persimmons, lotus leaves, lily bulbs, mung beans, pork skin, and sea cucumbers.

- **Foods belonging to the liver meridian:** Most *sour-tasting* and *green-colored* foods correspond to the liver meridian. These include tomatoes, papaya, hawthorn fruit, mulberries, cherries, loquat, plums, figs, sour dates, goji berries, dandelion, lotus leaves, chives, *Artemisia*, and bok choy.

- **Foods belonging to the spleen meridian**: *Sweet-tasting* and *brown-colored* foods correspond to the spleen meridian. these include fruits, all kinds of grains, beans, nuts, and most meats.

- **Foods belonging to the lung meridian:** Most *pungent* and *white-colored* foods correspond to the lung meridian, such as ginger, cilantro, onions, green onions, mustard seeds, turnip seeds, lotus, garlic, Sichuan peppers, water chestnuts, apricot kernels, lily bulbs, goat milk, and tangerine peel.

- **Foods belonging to the kidney meridian:** Most *salty* and *black-colored* foods correspond to the kidney meridians. Since the kidneys are related to longevity, aging, and well-being, eating dark-colored foods in our daily diet is part of the practice of promoting longevity. These include blueberries, blackberries, black beans, black rice, black sesame seeds, and dark-colored fruits and grains. As mentioned before, food that transforms more heaven-energy (sunlight) into its own storage as a plant or food, gives it a darker color. Other foods that nourish the kidneys and/or belong to the kidney meridian include garlic, chive seeds, wheat, fava beans, millet, wheat, kelp, sea cucumbers, shrimp, lamb, pork, scallops, goji berries, walnuts, grapes, lotus seeds, and cinnamon. The best black food is black ants!

- **Food belonging to the stomach meridian, paired with Spleen:** Ginger, green onions, bitter melon, Napa cabbage, celery, cucumbers, millet, sweet rice, buckwheat, apples, watermelon, hawthorn fruit, peaches, cherries, fiber nuts, barley, pork, and organic beef.

- **Food belonging to the urinary (bladder) meridian, paired with Kidney:** Corn, watermelon, winter melon, fennel, snow beans, snails, and cinnamon.

- **Food belonging to the large intestinal meridian, paired with Lung**: Potatoes, spinach, Napa cabbage, bitter melon, snow beans, bamboo shoots, mushrooms, soybeans, corn, honey, apricot kernels, bananas, figs, and pumpkin seeds.

- **Food belonging to the small intestinal meridian, paired with Heart:** Red beans, winter melon, cucumber, goat milk, and salt.

The Energy Direction of Food

The energy direction of food is very closely related to the temperature (Qi) and flavor of the food.

- **Yang food**: Warm and hot foods, with a pungent and sweet taste, belong to the yang food category; the energy direction of yang food is *upward*.

- **Yin food**: Cool and cold foods, with a sour, bitter, and salty taste, belong to the yin food category; the energy direction of yin food is *downward*.

In our daily lives, there are more foods that move energy downward (such as bitter-tasting foods, which can drain the body energy) than upward (such as sweet foods, which provide an instant upward-yang energy).

The Tonifying and Sedating Functions of Food

When we talk about the tonifying and sedating functions of food, we mean that we must *supplement the deficiency as a means to tonify*, and *reduce the excess as a means to sedate*. Tonifying and sedating are the two main functions of food.

Under these two main functions, TCM classifies food into several additional functions:

- **Functions of tonifying food**: tonifies energy (Qi), tonifies blood, tonifies yin, tonifies fluid, and tonifies Jing (essence).

- **Functions of sedating food**: disperses the surface (promotes sweating), opens orifices, releases heat, drains dampness, functions as a diuretic, clears fire toxins, functions as a laxative, and invigorates the body's Qi and blood.

- **Organs that tonify:** TCM has a long history of using animal organs to tonify or treat the same corresponding organ in humans, such as using the pancreas of pigs to treat diabetes, and using animal bone soup to tonify human bones. Pieces of the thymus, adrenal glands, and thyroid are used to treat endocrine disease, and the powder/energy from other animal organs are used in treating the same organs in humans. While there is some controversy and skepticism regarding this practice in modern society, in fact we are actually doing the same thing today. We simply use processed or artificial, synthetic forms of a "natural" substance rather than the whole, because of a scientific application more acceptable to the public and because people can more easily accept the idea of a scientific process.

Chapter 4
The Basic Concepts of Yao Shan and its Function

Yao Shan (*Yao* – medicinal spices and herbs; *Shan* – food cooked or prepared as a meal) has a long history in the legendary stories of China, an indication of humans having explored and experienced the various benefits of natural foods and plants (herbs) since ancient times. Until around the period of the Zhou dynasty (1000 BC), Chinese medical doctors who worked inside the palace were divided into one of four specialties, one of the four being a Yao Shan specialist. Yao Shan became one of the sophisticated trends in medicine that integrated medicinal herbs into food, with a specific way of preparing food with a good taste, color, and specific properties to promote the emperor's well-being, physical performance, longevity, and the prevention of diseases.

Inner Classic states that herbs and food come from the same source (having the same properties) and the different tastes of foods have different medicinal nutrients that balance different organs. This is why the Chinese call food therapy "Yao Shan" – *Yao*, medicinal herbs and spices, and *Shan*, food in general, prepared to best provide nutrients to the body, strengthen energy, nourish organs, improve circulation, detoxify the body, and support immunity. At the same time, not eating the right food according to one's physical condition might be detrimental to one's health.

A Chinese medicinal diet is not a simple combination of food and herbs, but a specially prepared dish made from Chinese herbs, certain foods, and condiments according to theoretical guidelines on the properties of the food and the way it should be prepared. Such a diet is in response to the different symptoms of disease and its diagnosis according to TCM, and is used to prevent and treat disease, improve well-being, enhance immunity, and slow down the aging process. At the same time, the body's physical condition changes according to different life stages, seasonal changes, and health status changes. The diet should be modified accordingly to assist the body in restoring its normal health status and to ensure free-flow of vital Qi (energy).

The Specific Characteristics of Chinese Yao Shan

TCM food therapy is based on the medical theory of TCM, of the balance of yin and yang and the five elements. According to the patient's constitution and patterns diagnosis, a specific food therapy is formulated by properly utilizing/assessing the different temperatures, colors, flavors, and tonic (or draining) properties of foods. In order to make a TCM diagnosis for an individual, a Chinese medical doctor has to understand the health condition and constitution of the individual in general, the condition and stage of the illness, and the seasonal considerations and changes according to geographic location. The doctor may then formulate the Yao Shan as it applies to that particular individual's condition. For example, a patient with a chronic, cold type of gastritis should be instructed to eat a certain kind of grain soup with warm herbs, such as dry ginger and cinnamon bark. A patient with menopausal syndrome, a yin deficiency resulting in feeling warm with hot flashes, should avoid hot, spicy food and add more cooling herbs to her diet, such as a tea made with chrysanthemum flowers, and goji berries added to a recipe for black rice soup.

Another common condition that people can self-treat with Yao Shan is digestive system weakness (spleen deficiency). A person manifests with low spirits, limb weakness, loss of appetite, and abdominal distension and cramps. First of all, it is important to avoid cold, raw, and greasy foods that will continue to weaken the energy in the digestive system. Rice soup should be made, with herbs such as Chinese red dates, ginger, Chinese yam, and ginseng, to restore and strengthen spleen function.

The fundamental aspect of TCM food therapy is to nourish Qi, blood, and body essence. Qi and blood are the basic materials for the body and organs to function. Essence is the most refined and fundamental substance for the body. However, the essence that the body acquired since birth, called pre-heaven essence, needs to continue to be replenished and nourished with a proper diet. In particular, those individuals who were born with a weak stomach or weak lungs (such as those with childhood asthma) should integrate Chinese food therapy as a lifestyle in order to continue to nourish and strengthen those organs, to prevent disease in a natural way and to treat the root causes, rather than passively doing nothing, only to have more health problems later in life. There are many natural foods to nourish the blood: dates, longan, lychee, sesame seeds, chicken liver, and chicken blood. Fruits that nourish body fluids include sugar cane, pears, water chestnuts, and watermelon. Deer meat and turtle meat nourish the body essence.

The key to Chinese food therapy is supporting and balancing the organs. The key to wellness and longevity is to balance the organs and the body, the mind, and the spirit. This does not mean that everyone needs to tonify, or that everyone needs to detoxify, without regard to individual body and organ conditions. If there is excess, there is no need to continue to tonify. If the body is accumulating toxins because it is too weak to expel them, one should strengthen the body with gentle, natural means in order to empower or restore the body's own Qi to detoxify itself, rather than utilizing harsh detoxifying methods—colonics or purging methods—which sometimes just do the opposite.

The basic principle is this: TCM food therapy is formulated according to the different patterns of each individual in order to facilitate and support the body's natural capacity. There is no one universal form or method for everything and everyone.

Believe that our body has its own capacity to heal itself. Whatever we do, we have to work with our body to facilitate it by following its natural path for healing. Even the greatest healer on the planet cannot revive the health of someone who has no desire or capacity to heal; trying to force the body against its own biological rhythm will not succeed.

TCM food therapy is a form of art. Prepared dishes should have attractive colors, smells, tastes, and designs. The formulation of a food therapy diet follows the same principle as when a TCM doctor writes a prescription for herbs, which is also an art form (there is the chief herb, the deputy herb, assistant herbs, and convoy herbs that work together like a battalion on the battle field). This means that the TCM doctor prepares the TCM food therapy not only for its therapeutic effect, but also considers the way to prepare, considering color, taste, body condition, the seasons—just like an art form. There are thousands of dishes, soups, congees, desserts, and herbal wines, and hundreds of books through the different dynasties, up until today. TCM food therapy is a specialty within the whole of TCM.

In general, foods that help promote well-being and increase body immunity are considered to be anti-aging foods, such as black sesame seeds, mulberries, wolfberries (goji berries), longan fruit, black walnuts, Chinese yams, Chinese red dates, grapes, lily bulbs, ginger, and pearl barley.

The Functions of TCM Food Therapy

1) Strengthening and Nourishing the Body Constitution

Food provides fundamental nutrition to all living things through the Three Treasures, Jing (essence), Qi (energy), and Shen (spirit). According to the different flavors of food, the nutrients of each flavor will nourish different organs. As mentioned previously, there are five flavors of food that enter five different organs accordingly.

Sour food enters the liver first; sweet food enters the spleen; pungent food the lungs; and salty food the kidneys. Different colors of foods have a tendency to enter certain meridians and their related organs. For example, tea (green color) tends to go to the liver meridian, pear (white color) to the lungs, rice (brown color) to the spleen and stomach, and black beans to the kidneys.

2) Nourishing the Body Essence, Nourishing Qi, and Supporting Shen

The design of TCM food therapy is based upon the classification of each kind of food's properties of nourishing, sedating, and balancing the condition of the body. Therefore, TCM food therapy can be used for the following:

<u>Nourishing the Body Essence</u>: Some of us were born with certain organ deficiencies or different body constitutions; that is why one person may have had childhood asthma (kidney deficiency that is not in harmony with the lungs), while another may have been a child with many gastrointestinal complaints and hyperactivity due to spleen deficiency that does not properly nourish the heart. Food therapy to strengthen the organs, beginning in childhood, is one of most common prevention treatments for childhood problems in TCM. It not only treats the childhood disease, but more importantly, it prevents health problems in adulthood that are related to the weak organ later in life. (The spleen-deficient child tends to gain weight in adulthood; the asthmatic child, if the asthma is related to the kidneys, tends to have fear, back problems, allergies, and low sexual drive later in life). When the TCM doctor asks a patient for their medical history, including childhood health problems, it will lead to the exploration of the adult disorder in order to develop the appropriate herbal and food therapy. For example, a patient who has complained of asthma since childhood may now be an adult with kidney deficiency problems, low back pain, and/or prematurely grey hair and low sex drive.

Nourishing Qi: The body's energy is dramatically depleted after chemotherapy, surgical procedures, childbirth, and chronic disease. Food therapy is commonly used to revive and strengthen the body's energy, restore the function of the vital organs, and restore the body's immunity (defensive system). Food therapy is most beneficial for recovering Qi in chronic conditions, alone or when combined with other treatments.

Supporting Shen: The spirits and emotions reflect each organ's energy. When the body and organs are harmonized, Shen (spirits and emotions) will be balanced and within normal boundaries. Healthy Shen reflects the organ's well-being. If an organ is in disharmony, the emotion related to that organ will be imbalanced. (The emotion related to the liver is anger; spleen is worry; heart is joy; kidney is fear; and lungs are sadness.) At the same time, obsession with or overindulgence in an emotion can have an impact on the related organ. TCM food therapy can play a part in overall well-being and treatment for emotional support. Sometimes we crave certain foods because of certain organ deficiencies; in another words, we will crave the taste that is related to the deficient organ. For example, when an elderly person has a kidney deficiency, osteoporosis, and back and knee weakness, they will tend to crave salty foods and have an element of fear in their emotional makeup, as these are the tastes and emotions related to the kidneys.

3) Treating and Preventing Diseases

TCM food therapy can help strengthen the deficient organ and balance the body's energy, nourish the blood, and normalize metabolism. Historically, TCM used fresh vegetables to treat scurvy, animal liver to treat night blindness, and kelp to treat thyroid problems. At the same time, the same food was used to prevent those diseases. There are many foods we eat every day that have therapeutic effects; we just need to know when to eat them more in order to prevent disease. For example, traditionally, mung bean was used as a soup for the prevention of summer heat stroke, and for cleansing the toxins in the body. Garlic should be eaten when the common cold is going around, as well as diarrhea. Green onions (the white part), ginger, and garlic soup should be eaten for the prevention and treatment of the early stages of a cold.

4) Promoting Anti-Aging and Well-Being (Longevity)

We should understand the word "longevity." It means that we can do whatever we can to delay the process of aging, but no one can stop the aging process, because aging is one of the laws of nature. But what we can do is to live healthier lives and enjoy life more, not suffering much disease or pain or becoming dependent as we age.

TCM food therapy is not the only answer to delay aging, but we should be aware of which food combinations can benefit us more. In the Qing dynasty, Dr. Chao Tin Dong, a longevity specialist, mentions *congee* for the promotion of well-being and the delay of aging. He stated, "When the elderly reach the golden age, they should eat congee several times a day or whenever they feel hungry to live a long life." There are hundreds of recipes for congee available in his book.

Throughout the long history of observation and practice, TCM has taught that certain foods have the property to promote well-being and should be considered to be anti-aging, or to delay aging. Some examples of these foods are sesame seeds, mulberries, longan, goji berries, black walnuts, royal jelly, Chinese wild yams, human milk, ginger, mushrooms, black/white fungus, tea, seaweed and kelp, and certain meats.

Chapter 5
How to Apply Food Therapy According to Age

Traditional Chinese Medicine (TCM) teaches that the body's function is to generate, maintain, protect, and repair the organs, including the sense organs, bones, and soft tissue throughout life. However, the balance among those organs' functions changes as we age. The more we physically or emotionally over-exert the body's capacity to repair itself, the more the body is out of balance and will deteriorate more quickly than it would through the natural aging process. Pursuing the goal of lifelong wellness requires us to adjust and match our nutritional intake in accordance with our age group. All food provided by our Mother Earth possesses unique properties with specific nutritional value. Some foods are blood-builders, others are brain foods, and others are muscle foods, while the rest may be energy foods. To support our life, which is composed of the Three Treasures—mind, body, and spirit—it is in our best interests to have a wide selection of food choices that we continually rotate from the vast variety provided by nature.

To stay healthy, one should eat according to one's age and physical needs. A diet that does not provide adequate nutrition to support the physical demands made on it, or is in excess of what the body needs, is harmful and could lead to serious health problems. Eating three meals a day at fixed times, in moderation, and with lots of variety, is recommended.

Yang Sheng in Childhood

Childhood Physiology Characteristics for Under Age 12

A child's body is young, active, and growing, both physically and mentally. Physically, children have tender and delicate organs, skin, and bone structure, and relatively weak defensive systems. They are sensitive to external environmental changes that cause yin-yang imbalance, because their bodies are not yet fully developed. During this time of rapid growth and development, yang-Qi dominates, creating a state of relative yin deficiency. This relative yin deficiency causes young children to have a tendency to suffer dehydration and electrolyte imbalance from over-heating, as well as vomiting and diarrhea. Dehydration in young children can quickly lead to a very dangerous condition.

Since young children's bodies demand a lot of nutrition to support growth, a strong spleen/digestive system is needed for this age group. However, the digestive system is still relatively delicate and weak, which is why young children tend to have digestive system (spleen) deficiency. According to TCM theory, spleen energy supports lung energy and the immune system. Once young children have a digestion issue, they are subsequently prone to catch colds and have ear infections and respiratory system disease due to the low lung energy that results from not having sufficient spleen energy support.

Psychologically, young children are emotionally dependent, unstable, sensitive, fearful, and easily intimated. Being treated with hostility and suffering emotional neglect often have a negative impact, not only psychologically in the short term, but also in long-term physical development and in the form of organ imbalances, with organ-related emotional disorders that can extend into the adult years.

Characteristic Diet Therapy for Childhood
- Avoid a restrictive vegetarian diet during childhood
- Eat more cooked, warm, easily digested food
- Avoid stimulating drinks such as coffee, soda, tea, alcohol, and any beverage containing artificial color, caffeine, or preservatives
- Avoid fried food

The Kidney Organs: TCM believes that the kidney organs are related to human development, bone structure, marrow, brain, and sexual organ development. During childhood, a diet with protein, animal liver, kidneys, and bone marrow (such as homemade bone soup) are very important for this age group. Other foods that nourish the kidneys are walnuts, black sesame seeds, mulberries, black beans, and other black-colored food.

Since this age group has more yang energy in the body, protein coming from fish, beans, eggs, pork, and milk is better than protein from "hot" foods like lamb, goat, ham, and sea cucumber. Just keep in mind that balance is key. "Hot" foods can be eaten, but not in excess, and not in the winter season.

The Spleen and Stomach Organs: In childhood, the spleen and stomach are still weak and prone to disorders when under physical and/or psychological stress. This is why children are susceptible to digestive problems such as abdominal cramps, vomiting, diarrhea, and parasitic disease, which lead to subsequent weakening of the immune and respiratory systems. In order to prevent digestive system disorders in childhood, it is important to control overeating and eating too much cold and raw foods, which continue to consume the energy of the spleen/stomach (digestive system). Instead, eat warm, cooked, soft foods that are easily digested and absorbed. From my observation in my practice, there is a high percentage of children with ear and repeat upper-respiratory infections that are not alleviated by multiple rounds of antibiotic treatment. Frequently, the infections recur, since the antibiotics further disrupt or damage the spleen/stomach energy, leading to diarrhea and malabsorption, which then further weakens the body's immunity. When a child exhibiting these problems sees a TCM doctor, the main strategy is to restore the child's digestive system and strengthen the spleen/stomach and lung organs with an herbal formula or simple food therapy, as well as pediatric Tui Na therapy (a special pediatric acupressure). This brings amazing results, without the need for continued use of antibiotics to treat chronic infection.

Several years ago, a young couple brought a six-month-old baby girl to our clinic. This young family had a very healthy diet and lifestyle. Both parents ate only organic, vegetarian, and mostly raw food. Apparently, the mother did not eat enough protein to produce milk for the baby, and the parents had been feeding their six-month-old a vegetarian diet of raw vegetable juice, or sometimes steamed vegetables. The baby looked malnourished, with dry skin and thin hair, and frequently suffered ear infections and diarrhea. Two rounds of antibiotics had only made the diarrhea worse. After speaking with and educating the young couple, we agreed to change the baby's diet to cooked, warm, pasty, and easily-digested food, along with pediatric Tui Na two to three times per day, to be conducted by the parents at home. With this simple food therapy, the baby quickly recovered.

A well-known Chinese idiom says, "If you want your children healthy and well, don't let them eat too much or be overly warm." TCM holds this to be the basic principle for small children's diets. There is training in cold resistance to enable children to better tolerate cold temperatures and enhance circulation of the blood and Qi (vital energy) to the body's surface so that it can defend against sickness. The stomach and intestines should not be overly filled; otherwise, undigested food easily turns into "evils," internal pathogens such as *heat evils*, *phlegm*, or *static fluid*, which can block the energy flow and function of organs and lower immunity. Proper diet can prevent the onset of disease, in addition to promoting growth and development, and is therefore vital during childhood.

A good rule of thumb is that all food should be easily digested. Fish, lean meats, soups, dairy products, eggs, and vegetables are all suitable. The body is developing healthy bones and muscles and requires a diet rich in protein and calcium. Children are very active and should eat regularly to maintain high energy levels. In contrast, over-consumption of sweet, fried, and greasy foods is not advised, since these cannot be digested properly. Instead, TCM teaches that these foods cause more heat and heat-related pathogens inside the body, such as fire and production of phlegm. Coffee, tea, spicy food, and, of course, liquors, should be prohibited.

Yang Sheng in Adolescence

Physiological Characteristics of Adolescents

Adolescence (12-18 years of age, or even extending to age 24) continues to be a period of active growth and rapid development, especially of the sex organs. According to TCM, during puberty the kidneys secrete a substance for promoting sex function, which is called *tian-gui*, from the abundance of stored kidney essence. As a result, a male will produce sperm, and a female will begin menstruation, signaling that the sex organs are mature and capable of reproduction.

Adolescence is the fastest stage of development in human life, with rapid physical changes, high energy, excellent memory and very active learning, creativity, sports activity, quick mood changes and emotionality, rebelliousness, and a tendency to be more independent, yet accompanied by much confu-

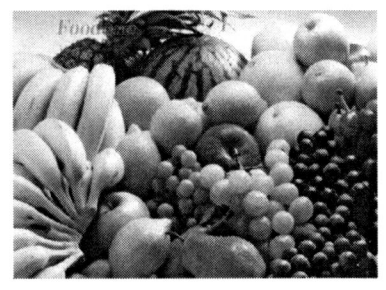

Banana, crab, lettuce, and watermelon are cold in energy.

sion. This is a very important, yet fragile, stage in psychological development. There are many factors that can impact an adolescent's physical and psychological development, such as the socio-economic environment, media influence, cultural values, community activity, education at school, parents and other role models, participation in after-school programs, and peer pressure.

Characteristic Diet Therapy for the Adolescent

At the adolescent stage, body mass increases, the organs develop, and metabolism is fast-paced. In particular, for the sexual organs to mature, there is a demand for more nutrients.

1. The body needs more proteins and carbohydrates, with a normal amount of fat.
2. The young male should avoid overeating and drinking.
3. The young female should emphasize a balanced nutritional diet, rather than consuming fast food or obsessively losing weight, leading to eating disorders.
4. If the adolescent has health problems, nutrition and diet therapy are even more important at this stage, to avoid many health problems later in life.
5. Developing a healthy lifestyle, good hygiene, a regular bedtime, and a diet and exercise program to change unhealthy habits all help to lay a good, healthy foundation for the future.

Adolescents should increase their daily intake of protein for rapid development. Consuming more fish, eggs, red meat, walnuts, and beans will tonify the kidneys, replenish marrow, and strengthen kidney energy for assisting sexual organ development. In other words, adolescents require good quantities of food in a well-balanced diet, with lots of calories and nutrients to support their development. Fresh, germinating vegetables, such as bean sprouts or bamboo shoots, are great for this age group, as are spicy and sour-tasting foods. Adolescents should avoid all stimulating drinks such as strong tea, coffee, commercial energy drinks (which are all sugar and caffeine), and alcohol. Besides the fact that these drinks stimulate the body to break down more nutrients and vitamins, in Chinese medicine it is believed that they belong to the "heat-generating substance" category of food that can cause heat in the stomach and skin problem such as acne. More heat in the body originating from an unhealthy diet can cause more "fire" emotions and the consumption of the body's kidney energy. In the short term, these beverages can make the adolescent more anxious, and can cause radical mood changes and sleeping disturbances. In the long term, if the kidney energy is exhausted, they can cause health problems such as insomnia, hypertension, heart problems, bone structure problems, and even infertility later in life.

Yang Sheng in Adulthood

Physiological Characteristics of Adulthood

This age group ranges approximately from age 25 to 36. At this stage of life, body growth ceases and/or has stopped. Body constitution is fully developed, having reached its strongest point, and Qi and blood are vigorous. The body has reached its optimal balance. However, this is the time when both sexes face many challenges and conflicts in life, such as establishing a relationship and family, focusing on a career, working hard, as well as enjoying life. The desire to be successful, and the "make more now to be better off later" mentality may drive and stress people at this stage of adulthood. Stressors from all sources impacting health, both physically and emotionally, can be a predominant factor in this age group, up until middle age.

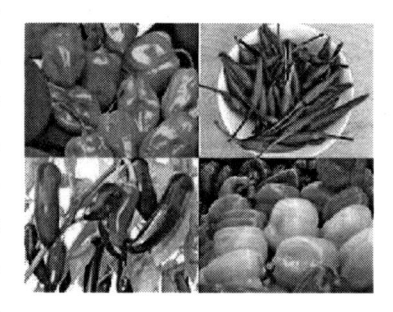

Pepper. Chile peppers are hot in energy.

Characteristic Diet Therapy for the Adult Group

Diet in this age group can include great variety, though a balanced diet should be the main focus. Those who have a high level of physical exertion in their profession, such as athletes, farmers, fishermen, or construction workers should eat more—especially carbohydrates—to maintain the immediate energy demands of the body. At the same time, the diet should be balanced, with protein and fat included. Both physical work and high metabolism can generate metabolic waste from the high levels of protein and fat in the body. In TCM, metabolic waste is called "heat" or "toxins," or it is identified by some as high acidity. To balance or neutralize the heat and detoxify the body, one should eat more vegetables and drink more green tea and fresh vegetable juice, since these are alkaline foods that can balance the heat/acidity of the body.

According to the concepts of bio-medicine, those in professions requiring a high level of intellectual work should consume a protein-rich diet to feed the brain. In Chinese medicine, the brain and bone marrow are ruled by the kidneys, and the "thought process" involves the spleen organ, too. Therefore, the diet should focus on strengthening both the kidneys and the spleen organ to avoid phlegm production, which leads to cloudy-mindedness.

Diet therapy in this age group should be modified according to body constitution type (see Chapter 7), seasonal changes, and profession. For example, a person with a yang body constitution should eat more yin (cold or cool) food. If this person continually eats too much hot or warm food, or follows an extreme diet of some sort that contradicts their body constitution type, it can lead to health problems. The body may begin to display an aversion to certain foods, or overreact and no longer be compatible with foods that were previously consumed with no problem. In bio-medicine, this is called a food allergy. For this reason, the TCM doctor will treat a patient with allergies by frequently monitoring diet, and balancing and strengthening the body so that it can recover its capacity, or energy, to process and accept the problem foods once again.

Many years ago, I had an out-of-state patient whose son made an appointment for him and flew him to San Diego. When I first met the patient, a tall, middle-aged gentleman, I was shocked by how thin he was. He had lost nearly all of his muscle, to the point of looking emaciated, like a skeleton. His skin was sallow, yellow, and dry, and he displayed a highly agitated emotional state. The patient's condition had been continually deteriorating for months, with no medical explanation, after having exhausted all nature of tests. Basically, the patient's diet did not fit his body constitution. The body had started to reject, or be allergic to, any kind of grain after he had eaten it for a couple of months. He would eat one grain, then switch to another type of grain for a couple of months, until there was nothing more he could eat, so he began to consume just a small amount of alcohol to get by. This is an extreme case of food incompatibility, with the spleen being too weak to process any food. We simply started with a very small amount of herb decoction to strengthen the spleen and stomach. Within several months, the patient resumed the ability to consume rice, wheat, and corn. He then gradually returned to normalcy.

Yang Sheng in Middle Age

Physiological Characteristics of the Middle-Aged Group

Middle age ranges from approximately age 36 to 60. Physically, the turning point of aging starts with this age group. Even though the organs and body meridians are full of energy and more stabilized, they start to gradually show signs of aging. Facial skin starts to show spots and have less collagen, the hair starts to turn gray, and there is the tendency to sit more and move less due to

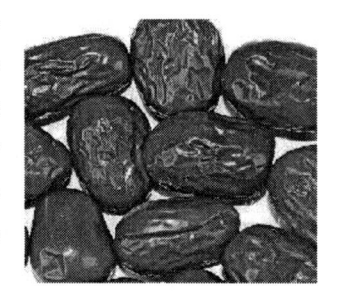

Chinese red dates have a tonifying property.

the body's tiring more quickly and having less endurance than in one's twenties and early thirties. Modern research indicates that after age thirty, human body function will reduce 1% for every year of age increase. The ancient TCM book *Inner Classic* states the same thing in the chapter titled "Heavenly Age": "Starting from the age of forty, the body's yin-Qi is only half left, and life activities start to slow down."

Even though most people in this age group are more emotionally and psychologically mature, they still have a hard time coping with the physical signs of aging, or are more paranoid about their own health and sensitive about age-related subjects. There is a saying in Chinese, "Middle age is the autumn full of events." This means that middle age is the autumn of life, with many stressors coming from social expectations and family, with children in college and aging parents. This is met with a body that has declining endurance and has begun to show other signs of aging. In this age group, if one has an unhealthy lifestyle—drinking, smoking, sleeping late, a fatty diet—one will age fast and suffer the many health problems that accompany premature aging.

Chinese medicine offers Yang Sheng to this age group, which is a critical stage for promoting well-being and longevity, and for preventing disease.

Yang Sheng Guidelines for Middle Age
1. *Calm the spirit and worry less.* Reducing stress and balancing the emotions is one of the most important ways to slow down the aging process. Middle age generally carries the most stress. The ancient book, *Record of Yang Sheng and Longevity*, states: "Middle-aged people should learn how to compete without the desire to win, and calm the spirit by emptying the mind of thought." It also teaches that during this period of life, one should develop more entertaining habits by pursuing interesting and relaxing activities, such as bird-watching or raising birds, painting, singing, dancing, and joining friends

for conversation and/or travel. Simply dressing up for social events can make one feel happy and younger.

2. *Avoid physical over-exertion.* The life of middle-aged people is like a sandwich, burdened with taking care of the younger and older generations. It can mean years of stress accumulation, lack of sleep, and being on-the-go all the time. Taking time for one's self by simply resting and sleeping more can be a simple but very rewarding way to rejuvenate the body and slow down aging. It may require one to better organize one's schedule in order to make time. Relaxation exercises like yoga, Tai Chi, and Qigong are good anti-aging activities.

3. *Restrain Sexuality.* TCM teaches that kidney energy controls aging, bone structure, and sexuality, and is housed in the lower back, opening in the ears. Overly indulging in sex, having multiple abortions, miscarriages, and/or childbirths very close together, or taking drugs to stimulate the body to force it to perform, are all activities that deplete the kidney's vital energy (or kidney essence). A person with depleted kidney essence has decreased sexuality, more weakness and pain in the lower back and legs, hearing loss at an early age, and bone structure problems—in a word, more signs of premature aging. Physical decline starts in middle age, so it is believed that restraining one's sexuality in order to preserve the kidneys for one's well-being in middle age is a very important Yang Sheng method. Throughout history, more emperors died at an early age because of overly indulging in sexual activity. Only a few emperors in Chinese history lived longer—those who totally restrained their sexual activity after age 50.

Clinically, we have seen many cases of young male patients who have sexual problems and signs of premature aging. After taking their personal history, we find that in most cases, they had a history of abusing drugs and herbs in order to force the body to perform sexually, exhausting the kidney essence and not giving the body time to recover its energy. In female patients, multiple miscarriages or childbirths close together do not give the body time to recover, causing it to lose its kidney essence. These patients also show signs of premature aging at a relatively young age. Restraining sexual activity and preserving more kidney energy can assist in the body's well-being and longevity and prevent the degenerative diseases of middle age. *Record of Yang Sheng and Longevity* advises, "People over 30, once every 8 days; over age 40, once every 16 days; and over age 50, once every 21 days, will allow the body to recover and not be overly exerted, but with modification depending on the weakness or strength of the individual's body constitution."

Characteristic Diet Therapy for the Middle-Aged Group

TCM teaches that signs of aging appear in middle-age. But active measures, such as with exercise or diet, can preserve health, delay the process of aging, and reduce the risk of chronic degenerative disease while laying a good foundation for old age. According to TCM, good nutrition plays a vital role in reducing health risks. Chinese medicinal food therapy is the optimal choice for this stage. However, one should consult a TCM doctor and herbalist to have a professional recommendation. Herbs of similar, supporting, or enhancing natures are added to food to intensify the body's functions. Special therapeutic diets are consumed regularly and frequently to nourish the body. All food therapies follow the guideline of specific body constitutions and are modified according to seasonal changes (refer to Chapters 6 and 7). These are designed to assist the body in healing itself, with comprehensive and permanent results. Some simple therapeutic recipes have become popular family dishes and delicacies in Chinese cuisine. Examples of common anti-aging foods are royal jelly, pollen, legumes, mushrooms, white fungus, carp, black sesame seeds, walnuts, bamboo shoots, black figs, black mulberries, Chinese red dates, and pine nuts.

Yang Sheng for the Elderly

<u>The Physiological Characteristics of the Elderly</u>
This age group is considered to be aged 60 and older. By now, we understand that TCM teaches that throughout one's entire life span, kidney essence is the master of development, bone structure, and productivity, opening in the ears. Kidney energy, as with the other organs, abides by the law of natural aging. This organ's energy decline is a normal aging process, called "physiological deficiency" in TCM. This compares a healthy 60-year-old with him/herself at the age of 20. However, if a 20- or 30-year-old has the physical endurance and function of a 50- or 60-year-old body, it is out of balance and called "pathologically deficient." This indicates the need for professional help in order to restore the body's normal function, according to its age.

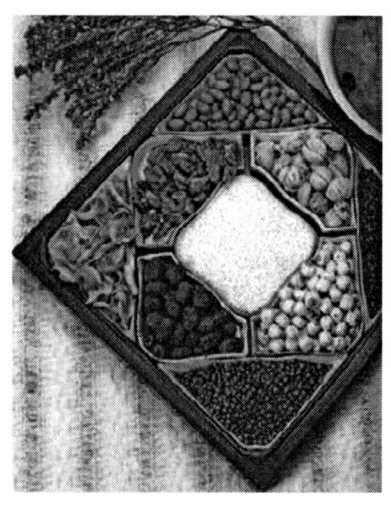

Walnut, Chinese red date, black beans, lily bulb, and lotus seeds are good for the elderly.

TCM believes that the amount of stored kidney essence dictates the speed of the natural process of aging. If one can store significant amounts of kidney essence, one can live longer and be healthier. Kidney essence comes principally from one's parents at birth. If they were young, healthy, and carrying strong family genes when conceiving, then they will pass on strong kidney essence. However, lifestyle is also a factor in preserving kidney essence as we become older. It can be compared to a person who inherits a set amount of money at birth. On the one hand, the more money inherited, the longer one may live. On the other hand, regardless of how much money one may inherit, if one is careless and spends mindlessly, even a large amount will not last long. In the same way, unfortunately, kidney essence is very hard for the body to make after birth. But by modifying our lifestyles and balancing ourselves physically and mentally, we can preserve it to live longer and healthier lives. This is the key meaning of *yang sheng*: nourishing life.

In old age, when the manifestations of aging appear, such as loose teeth, hair loss, and stiffness in the joints, bones, and tendons, this means the organs are under-functioning, and the Qi, blood, and body fluids are inadequate.

When the body becomes weak, adaptation to environmental change is slow. When social or economic conditions change, some older people become more isolated and have limited physical activity, which then leads to emotional and psychological changes, such as sadness, depression, and impatience, or even distrust and paranoia.

Yang Sheng Guidelines for the Elderly
1. **No pretensions or high expectations.** Being happy with what one has—being generous and helping others—are virtues that can promote well-being and longevity, as stated in the book *The Wisdom of Preserving Essence and Longevity*. Older people can share their vast life experience and wisdom with others; restrain desires; keep young at heart, without losing a sense of reality; love life; and keep the brain active by reading, attending school, group activities, or participating in community volunteer work.
2. **Avoid unhealthy and negative environments and events.** Year after year, some of our elderly friends will go to another world. Especially for those older people who are already emotionally sensitive, this can bring a feeling of negativity and fear. *The New Book of Nourishing Life for the Elderly*, from the Song dynasty, states that the family should assist the elderly by not attending funerals; avoiding the scenes of disastrous

events or where a murder might have occurred; not showing panic and sadness in front of an ill elderly person; not predicting or reporting bad news; not allowing the elderly to live alone in an environment without sun and proper hygiene; not allowing the elderly to meet with unwanted persons; and, for the older person's well-being, creating a good, positive environment and living conditions that foster happiness, confidence, and emotional balance. There is a saying in our society: "Mind over body." For both mental and physical health, maintaining positive thoughts seems to be even more important for this age group.

3. **Regular sleep; gentle movements; and taking anti-aging safety measures**. As part of normal aging, the elderly have Qi and blood deficiencies. With declining body energy, blood circulation will slow down; with a declining defense/immune system, the body is more prone to catching cold or cold-related diseases and having arthritis and body pain. There is a saying in Chinese medicine: "Blood flows to where the Qi (energy) goes." It is important to get enough sleep and to nap during the daytime to rejuvenate the body, and to gently exercise, moving the body's Qi and blood to help maintain health. Many books in Chinese medical history point out that elderly people should sleep alone and refrain from sexual activity in order to ensure a good, restful sleep as an important anti-aging measure.

Characteristic Food Therapy for the Elderly

Good nutrition and diet therapy can be challenging for the elderly. As stated above, in old age, all organ functions decline, including the digestive system. The original Qi decreases, as does blood circulation, both of which comprise the body's defensive energy. This condition requires the support of proper nutrition. One challenge facing the elderly is a decrease in appetite and a lack of interest in food due to the decline of the senses of smell and taste, so that with advancing age, the amount of food intake decreases. Another challenge is that the digestive system becomes less efficient in the absorption of nutrients. These challenges can be addressed, however, if the physiological changes taking place with this age group are properly understood.

TCM food therapy can be applied to prevent the further depletion of kidney essence, to restore the body's Qi and blood, and most importantly, to harmonize and preserve spleen energy (the digestive system) to some degree. However, it takes much longer to restore and see the benefit of any therapies in the elderly. Therefore, it is important to be patient and persistent and choose a more natural way of healing. Older people should eat small, easily digested meals, but more frequently throughout the day. The food should be cooked and soft, easy to digest and absorb. Congee (porridge) is one of the best choices for this age group. There are a variety of congee therapies for the variety of conditions found in the elderly.

Congee has traditionally been used as a natural healing food therapy in the Chinese culture for different age groups and their differing conditions. In modern China, one can find many congee restaurants in both big cities and remote areas.

Food categories suitable for the elderly are those that principally benefit Qi, promote blood production, and regulate the functioning of the organs. Food should be soft, bland, warm, and more liquid, or semi-liquid (pasty), for the more advanced in age. Some commonly used foods are Indian bread, Chinese wolfberries, black soybeans, water caltrop, Chinese dates, peaches, flax seeds, walnuts, grapes, and lotus seeds.

The following are some examples of food therapy for the elderly that promote well-being and longevity:

- **Longevity Five Bean Milk:** Soybeans, black beans, green beans, lima beans, and peanuts, in the ratio of 3:1:1:1:1. Soak overnight (6-12 hours) and use a soybean milk machine to make milk. This congee nourishes the liver and the kidneys; is anti-aging; increases immunity; lowers cholesterol and blood pressure; prevents coronary artery disease; and is good for diabetes.

- **Longevity Congee**: Sweet rice, black rice, black beans, mung beans, red beans, barley, buckwheat, walnuts, peanuts, goji berries, sunflower seeds, black sesame seeds, lotus seeds, and 5-7 Chinese red dates. Put in a crock pot with plenty of water and cook overnight (8-10 hours) or longer.

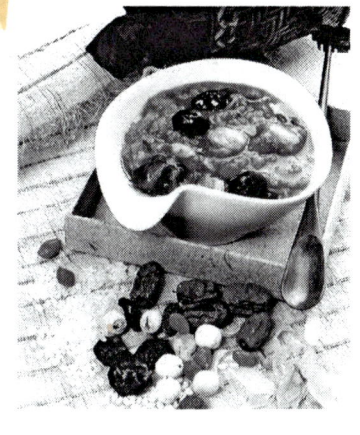

Longevity Congee

Yang Sheng for Pregnancy and Postpartum

Physiological Characteristics of Women

During their sexually productive years, women are a special group, with special physiological conditions and medical problems related to the menstrual cycle, pregnancy, giving birth, and nursing. At the same time, women in general express their feelings and emotions more freely, which can consume more of the body's Qi and blood energy and lead to more health problems.

Hygiene Concerns during Menstruation

During the menstrual period, TCM teaches that the woman's blood chamber (uterus) is open to the external environment, so that it is prone to invasion by cold pathogens, heat, and toxins (infectious agents). TCM doctors advise that during the menstrual cycle, women should be aware of the followings tips, in order to prevent health problems later in life:

a) Keep good hygiene habits: During the menstrual cycle, try to avoid bubble baths, swimming, and sexual activity, as well as certain kinds of ob/gyn check-ups. It is easy to understand that during the menstrual cycle, blood vessels in the uterus are open, and blood itself is a good medium for bacteria to grow. Avoid non-sterile water, liquid, and other objects that might introduce pathogens into the uterus and blood circulation system, causing infection. During the menstrual cycle, in order to have a smooth flow of blood without pain, TCM teaches that one should avoid contact with cold, such as walking in the rain, sitting on cold benches, or eating or drinking cold food and beverages. Cold causes contraction and closes the meridians and energy circulation in channels, leading not only to more menstrual cramping, but also to many cold-related problems in the long term, such as coldness and pain in the lower lumbar, knees, and limbs. Consistently coming into contact with cold during the menstrual cycle can be very harmful, leading to an infertility condition referred to as "cold womb syndrome."

TCM believes that blockage of the free flow of Qi and blood in the meridians, blood vessels, or inside an organ can cause pain. "If there is blockage, there is pain," is a common saying in TCM. However, there are many possible causes for a blockage, such as extreme cold or extreme heat that damages the fluid and meridians; deficiency of energy or blood so that there is not enough flow in the meridian channels; or a blockage from a reversal of the normal direction of energy flow in an organ.

Normally, there are two important meridians (the Chong and Ren meridians) related to the menstrual cycle, fertility, and pregnancy. If there is abundant blood and Qi and an even temperature, without extreme hot or cold, and there is no blockage, then there will be no premenstrual stress syndrome, cramps, or painful menstruation, and fewer problems with fertility. Sexual activity during the menstrual cycle will disturb the normal flow of the meridians and weaken kidney energy, while increasing the risk of contact with pathogens.

b) Maintain emotional balance: A well-balanced emotional state reflects physical well-being, and vice versa. TCM believes that obsessive thinking, pent-up emotions, and persistent worrying, sadness, and anger can compromise menstrual flow, causing menstrual disorders, a lackluster facial complexion, and fertility disorders. Repressed emotion can cause body Qi stagnation or Qi direction disorders, so that Qi cannot build blood flow. It is very common, clinically, to see women—especially career women working under high stress, or young college graduates who have moved to a new city or started new living or working conditions—who present with body stress and the tendency to have menstrual disorders and severe premenstrual syndrome (PMS). It is my observation that some women who have Qi/blood stagnation and very painful menses, who may be very emotional and have had many premenstrual symptoms for years without proper treatment, will tend to develop fibrosis years later if not treated. This is long-term Qi and blood stagnation, which causes the formation of lumps. Others are young patients who are on birth control pills because of their PMS; some are even taking anti-psychotic medication for their PMS. Not only does this medication not treat the root cause of the problem, but in some cases it makes it worse (a couple of my young patients became manic after taking birth control pills). It is important to understand how to work with the body naturally and follow its natural laws. If the body shows symptoms, there must be imbalance in the organs, either an underlying deficiency or an underlying excess. Acupuncture and an herbal formula—which balance the body and treat the cause, rather than merely masking the symptoms—are the optimal methods for reducing menstrual cycle-related stress and emotional disorders.

c) Maintain diet: After determining the root cause of the condition, if a woman has a lot of blood deficiency, she should consult a TCM doctor for food therapy and a blood-nourishing herbal formula. Blood is a vital substance for the body, especially for women because of their special physiological condition. During menses, each month a woman has to lose some blood; so to nourish blood energy, before or during the menstrual cycle, she should eat more nutritious food with more easily digested protein, whole grains, and plenty of orange- and green-vegetables. During the menstrual cycle, she should avoid hot, spicy, and pungent food, which causes more heat and consumes more blood energy (yin). At the same time, she should avoid the consumption of cold and raw food, which blocks and contracts the meridians, leading to painful menstruation and cramps, and can even stop menstrual flow.

Yang Sheng During Pregnancy (Yang Sheng starts with the fetus)

During the course of pregnancy, from conception until birth, proper nutrition and supplementation are fundamental for the protection and nourishment of the fetus. The health condition, nutritional status, and mental, emotional, and spiritual state of the mother during pregnancy all have a significant impact on the well-being of the child.

a) Fetus Education: There are many books in Chinese medical history that state that during pregnancy, a woman should act properly and speak no bad words; she should not be pretentious or jealous, or a witness to evil. Rather, she should help others with a spirit of generosity and goodwill, since the mother's good spirits will impact the fetus. She should also listen to beautiful music and go sight-seeing to beautiful places during her pregnancy, in order to be relaxed and feel happy, ensuring good Qi and harmonized blood, which assist in consolidating the essence of the fetus.

There are many books and wisdom from thousands of years of Chinese history indicating that the mother's good spirits during pregnancy will result in good energy (Qi) in the fetus. Some of these ancient books include elaborate details about how to cultivate a feeling of happiness and stimulate the five sense organs by looking at beautiful flowers or birds, such as peacocks, listening to the sound of a waterfalls and the singing of birds, and avoiding all evil Qi and unhappy events, such as funerals, throughout the course of the pregnancy.

b) Fetus Training: During the second trimester of the pregnancy, at the beginning of the thirteenth week, the fetus is completing its full development of the middle ear and the other sense organs. A mother should communicate with her fetus by talking, reading stories and poems, singing, and playing beautiful music to stimulate the fetus's senses. In Chinese culture, it is believed that a woman who laughs and smiles a lot during pregnancy will have a happy baby. Once a woman is pregnant, her colleagues and coworkers, neighbors, and even people she meets on the street always pay special attention to her, giving advice and support, and making good conversation that causes her to smile and laugh. The older people will always remind her that she will make her baby calm, happy, and healthy if she goes for a walk in the park to listen to the birds singing or to the sound of water. Not taking these measures can result in a less fortunate outcome, with a child that has a predisposition for hyperactivity disorder, a short attention span and inability to focus, and more anxiety and nervousness as he or she grows up.

One kind of training for the fetus is to gently massage it after 20 weeks of pregnancy. The best time to do this is before sleep, especially during the last trimester of pregnancy. This initiates and stimulates fetal movement. From clinical observation, it has been found that the fetus with this training will learn standing and walking much earlier than without this training. If the mother starts having contractions in the last trimester, however, this training is not recommended.

c) Sexual Activity during Pregnancy: Pregnant women should refrain from sexual activity during the first and last trimesters of pregnancy. TCM teaches that during the early stages of pregnancy, all the body's Qi and blood accumulate in the womb (at the Chong and Ren meridians) in order to nourish the fetus. This constitutes the body's defensive energy for the special condition of pregnancy. This is why a woman is prone to catch colds and get sick during the first trimester, since so much Qi and blood flows to the lower body to support the pregnancy. The digestive system's energy direction should go downward, but instead there is more stagnation, or even a reversal in direction upward, causing nausea and vomiting in this early stage.

If, during this first trimester, there is a lot of sexual activity, it will cause more Qi-flow disorder in the lower body, and the fetus's nourishing yin-Qi will leak out of the uterus, which can cause toxins to invade the uterus and result in miscarriage. Then, during the last trimester, especially in the last month before delivery, TCM teaches that too much sexual activity can cause premature delivery or difficulty in delivery, and the fetus will have a higher likelihood of being mentally retarded or having a lower IQ and more disease, including degenerative disease, at a young age. Some clinical observation and research notes that sexual activity in the month of delivery results in a higher infection and fetus mortality rate, a 68% higher probability of a lower IQ than the comparison group, and 100% higher rate of jaundice after delivery.

d) Food Therapy during Pregnancy: A proper diet during pregnancy not only supports and nourishes both the fetus and the mother, but builds a solid foundation for a healthy child after birth and a healthy postpartum for the mother.

In the first trimester (1-3 months), the woman should eat less than normal and add a little sour-tasting food to each meal to help soothe the appetite. She should try to avoid hot, spicy, and greasy food, since most women tend to have sensitive digestive systems and morning sickness during this time. Adding ginger to the diet and eating warm food to assist and calm digestion is recommended. In some cases, morning sickness can be resolved by simply drinking warm tea with fresh ginger (cut into small pieces) and honey.

During the second trimester of pregnancy (4-7 months), the woman should eat more protein and calcium-rich food, such as bone soup, milk, egg yolks, and leafy green vegetables. Phosphate-rich food can help the development of the brain and central nervous system, including soybeans, chicken, lamb, and egg yolks. There is more warmth in the uterus during the second trimester, so ingesting food with cooling properties—such as fresh fruit and vegetables—can balance the heat.

When the pregnancy has reached the third trimester (8-10 months), the fetus develops very fast, storing energy and nutrients in its body. This is a vital stage for brain development. During this stage, tonic foods such as eggs, seafood, meat, and beans are normally consumed regularly, but should be cut down in the final months before delivery to reduce the risk of a large baby and difficult birth. The woman should also reduce salt intake to prevent edema and hypertension related to the pregnancy. Hot and spicy food should also be avoided during this stage in order to eliminate excess heat; we sometimes see newborns with skin problems resulting from the mother's consumption of too much hot, spicy food during the pregnancy.

Throughout the entire pregnancy, the mother's diet and emotional state not only impact the fetus in pregnancy, but the lifelong well-being of the child. TCM believes that a strong, balanced body constitution comes from its " pre-heaven Qi," or "congenital essence," which refers to the period before one is born; the congenital essence of the fetus is cultivated and developed during pregnancy. If there is smoking, alcohol, and/or drug abuse during pregnancy, the child may have lifetime health problems, both physically and emotionally.

Another important fact is that pregnancy at an older age will run the same risk of weak congenital essence. According to TCM theory, congenital essence is kidney essence, and as we age, our kidney essence lessens (women start to decline in kidney essence at age 28). As kidney essence declines, there is not an adequate amount to support and to give to the fetus. As a result, there is a higher chance of mental retardation (such as Down Syndrome) and lower academic achievement, degenerative disease, immunity disorders, and emotional problems in adulthood. Similarly, if a woman has repeat miscarriages, abortions, and/or multiple pregnancies that are very close together, her body has no time to rejuvenate and restore the kidney essence, so she will not have enough kidney essence to give to and support the fetus in pregnancy. In my practice, there have been times when I could not explain why a patient had a degenerative disease at an early age, without a family history of disease or an unhealthy lifestyle. However, after checking, I would see a clear connection between the patient's mother's pregnancy history and my patient's problem. Along the same lines, particularly with academic achievement, it will be the oldest child of the family who outperforms the younger siblings.

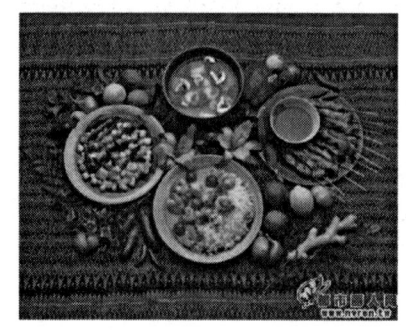

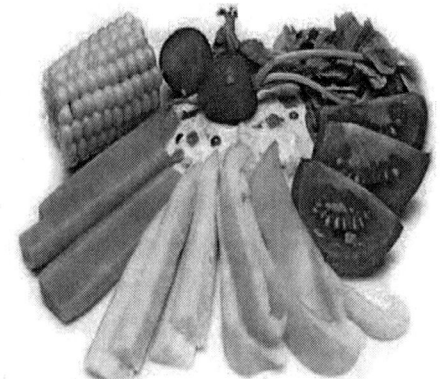

Examples of cooling foods: cucumbers, bean curd, radishes, and strawberries

Food Therapy in the Postpartum Period

Six to eight weeks after childbirth is considered to be a very critical period for both the mother and the newborn infant. "Labor" in childbirth derives its meaning from the extreme consumption and exhaustion of the mother's Qi and blood. The first twenty-four hours after labor, the woman must stay in bed to sleep and should consume only warm, nutritious liquid or semi-liquid food to nourish Qi and blood. Otherwise, the pelvic muscles cannot recover their strength, and the Qi will be unable to hold and guide the blood and keep the organs in their proper places, so that there will be hemorrhaging and a prolapsed uterus. When there is Qi deficiency after childbirth, the body has very weak defensive strength, especially the defensive energy that controls the skin and pores to fend off pathogens and cold and wind exposure. That is why the woman sweats excessively after giving birth, and is prone to cold and wind attack. Since there is blood deficiency, the organs are not being nourished adequately—especially the heart, liver, and spleen—and there is a greater propensity to have emotional problems such as sadness, depression, crying easily, and/or feeling fearful, depending on which organ deficiency is predominant.

Different cultures have different concepts and rules regarding what to do or not do during the first month after labor. In the TCM view, great precautions should be taken during the first month postpartum not to come into contact with cold, such as drinking cold water, eating cold food, or washing the hands with cold water; and avoiding places where the body is exposed to wind, especially after bathing, such as being in a car with the windows down. *Qian Jin Yao Fong*, written by the famous doctor Sun Si Miao about 2,000 years ago, states that after childbirth, the woman's Qi, blood, and five organs are all deficient. Therefore, the woman should rest for 100 days, get plenty of sleep, be sheltered from fear or emotional disturbances, and refrain from sexual activity. According to clinical observation, most women in the Chinese culture believe that body and joint pain can be lifetime problems if a woman is careless during the first month postpartum by coming into contact with the cold and exposing herself to the wind. In the first month postpartum, even just eating something cold one time, or using cold water to rinse the mouth, or standing a short while out on the patio and allowing the wind to blow on the neck, is enough to cause muscle pain for years. In Chinese culture, disease from the first month postpartum is called *yue zi bing* (first month postpartum disease). It is also believed that body and joint pain from this period can last for years, will always recur, and will be very difficult to totally eliminate.

Yang Sheng Methods during the Postpartum Period

a) Enough sleep, rest, and moderate movement: Sleep, sleep, and more sleep is one of the most important ways for the body to recover from exhaustion. Some women complain that they cannot sleep well during the first month postpartum. One piece of advice from the Chinese elders in this situation is: *When the baby sleeps, you sleep; when the baby eats, you eat.* Take the month off from any sort of work and your regular routine to just focus on yourself and your newborn. When the baby is asleep, the mother has time to sleep and rest in bed. When the baby wakes up and needs to eat, the mother can nurse the baby while drinking nutritious soup. If she drinks too much water, her milk will be too thin. Always have a big pot of nutritious soup slowly cooking, or ready and warm on the stove. Try not to eat too much solid food; it is not advisable to consume solid food right after labor because solid food uses more of the body's energy and is harder for the body to digest. The body can use liquid food right away to make milk for nursing. Another benefit is that the body will not normally gain weight from liquid food. There are a number of lactation-enhancing food therapies that Chinese families have been using for centuries that are beneficial to both mother and newborn. There is no food on this earth that is as good as mother's milk for the infant. I strongly recommend that women try food therapy to promote lactation.

b) Modified diet to increase nutrition: With depleted Qi and blood after labor, proper nutrition and diet are vital, and the mother must be sure to have sufficient nutrients for nursing. The digestive system is as strong as before labor, though it may be more sensitive. First, in order to preserve digestive system energy, the mother should not eat too much solid, cold, raw, or greasy food. If there is a digestive system disorder, not only will both mother and child suffer, but there will also be more health and weight problems later in life. Second, the mother should also avoid hot and spicy food that can cause fluid loss and constipation, and also bleeding. Finally, she should avoid overeating and feeling too full, or waiting too long between meals and feeling too hungry. The mother should eat smaller portions, four to six meals a day, just as the newborn baby eats many times per day.

For the first 1-3 days after labor, the mother should consume soup made with lean meat and eggs, or porridge (congee) made from rice or millet. Other soups she can consume are chicken soup, bone soup, whole grain congee with soy, and vegetable soup, which must be cooked until soft with ginger to protect the stomach. Also, the chicken in the chicken soup must be whole, organic chicken that is cooked for a long time until the meat and bones are falling apart and all the nutrients from the bones, cartilage, skin, collagen, and meat are fully absorbed into the soup broth.

By closely observing the newborn's skin reaction to her diet, the mother can discover whether it is a diet fit for the infant or not. For example, when the mother eats hot and spicy food, the baby may develop a face rash; if she uses a lot of salt, there may be white spots on the newborn's lips.

The following are some examples of food therapy for promoting the mother's health and lactation:

Pig's Feet Soup

Two whole large pig's feet
Raw peanuts: 200g
Green onions: 2 pieces
Ginger: 10g
Cooking wine: 2 tbsp
Salt

Combine all the ingredients together with water and cook for 2-4 hours until the soup becomes milky. Drink the broth only, or use the broth as stock for other vegetable or noodle soups.

Carp Tail Soup

One big carp tail: approx. 500g (1 lb)
Raw peanuts: 200g
Cooking wine (rice wine): 2 tbsp
Ginger: 10g

Cook ingredients in water until carp tail falls apart. Drink the broth only (no salt).

Chicken Soup

One whole organic chicken: approx. 500g
Dried lily flower (*huang hua cai*): 30g, soaked in water until soft
Ginger: 10g
Rice wine: 2 tbsp
Raw peanuts: 200g
Chinese red dates: 4 pieces
Pinch of salt

Cook all ingredients together with water in a big pot for 2-4 hours. Drink the broth, or use it as a base to make noodle and rice soups. More water can be added to continue cooking until the chicken meat and bones are falling apart. Drink the broth and eat the meat, if desired.

c) Hygiene: Following labor, there will be excessive perspiration, uterine bleeding, and labor-related wounds, so the mother should not take a bath for at least 4 weeks, but shower instead. She should take care of any wounds using sterilized gauze bandages. TCM teaches that she should refrain from sexual activity for 100 days (three months) following labor to avoid infection and to ensure a complete recovery. She must remember to wash her hands and clean her nipples before nursing. Utensils can be kept clean by simply boiling them in water, without detergent.

d) Eliminate medication while nursing: Many medications can be transmitted via the mother's breast milk, impacting the infant's health. The nursing mother must be very careful when taking any medications, supplements, or herbal formulas. It is best to try to eliminate all medications during this period to avoid causing infant intoxication. If at all possible, the mother should try to find alternative treatments to alleviate her health concerns while nursing.

<u>Yang Sheng during the Menopausal Period</u>

After age 45-50, women enter the menopausal period. This period marks the beginning of a slow process of change and is the stage of life when a woman goes from full maturity to the beginning of natural aging and naturally weakening productivity. The Chinese call menopause the *Geng Nian* period, meaning the "years of change." In Western cultures, a higher percentage of women suffer from clinical symptoms during this time than are found in Asian women. I would point out that this is not only because Asian women eat more tofu than Western women, as claimed by commercialized soy supplement companies. There is more to it than this. During this stage, kidney energy and its related meridians—the Chong and Ren meridians—start to show physiological deficiency, with weakening and a lack of blood. This is why the menstrual cycle becomes irregular and gradually stops. Blood is yin material in the body; when it naturally dries up, the balance between yin and yang is tilted. As a result, yang is in relative excess, with less yin to balance it out. The body will then manifest more false yang activities: heart palpitations, insomnia, nervousness, anxiety, hot flashes, headaches, and tinnitus—all the symptoms of menopausal syndrome. Once the cause of the problem is understood as a simple imbalance of yin and yang, menopausal syndrome can be overcome with food therapy and herbs with cooling properties to cool yang and nourish and strengthen yin. It is simple as taught in TCM, and it is simple in practice.

The notion that "hormone replacement therapy" is the only way to deal with menopausal syndrome is found only in Western cultures. A normal aging condition, menopausal syndrome has been with human beings since long before the concept of "hormones" was discovered less than 200 years ago. Different cultures always had natural ways of dealing with and treating what we now identify as menopausal syndrome, but as time has gone by, this has been overlooked or forgotten. Approximately forty years ago, doctors discovered that there were more cancers in women who had had hormone replacement therapy (HRT). I was shocked when I came to the United States twenty years ago and met so many people on HRT, after not having known anyone in China on HRT. As a matter of fact, I call using birth control pills—which contain hormones—"hormone interrupting therapy" (HIT). If a teenager starts using birth control pills, and then later begins HRT after menopause, then most of the woman's life is on HIT or HRT. There are no studies that have been conducted to show how HIT impacts women over the long term. Many women are confused or misled by so-called "bio-identical" hormones, thinking that it is not dangerous at all because they are almost like real human hormones. Very few women ask their doctors to disclose the truth about "bio-identical" hormones.

Before we can understand hormones, let's see how natural hormones in the body are related to life span and cell growth. Hormone secretion in the body is like anything else—it follows the laws of nature and the human biological clock cycles. From the very first day of life to the very last, and at each stage throughout the life cycle, our biological clock naturally programs the body to produce different hormones at the different stages of life. Hormones also stimulate the cells of target organs to proliferate, such as female sex hormones that stimulate the growth of the inner lining of the uterus and breast tissue. In this way, all the hormones stimulate their specific target organs to proliferate. Once cells are stimulated to proliferate and multiply, there is always the chance that the newly generated cells may be abnormal or deformed, may malfunction, or may even become cancerous. However, when we are young, we have strong immune cells such as CD4, CD8, and NK (natural killing) cells that recognize and eliminate abnormal cells, including cancerous cells. When we age, our body's biological clock naturally slows down or stops the secretion of hormones, along with the body's naturally weakening immune cells. This is how the body naturally stays in balance.

At the same time, we must understand that when we age, the aged cells will make more mistakes during proliferation. For this reason, when external hormones are introduced into the body at a time when the body should be naturally without them, there will be more production of abnormal or cancerous cells from the hormone stimulation, without the corresponding production of potent immune cells to defend the body from growing cancers. This will be the case, no matter how good a form of hormone we use. Or, perhaps we stored our own hormones during our youth, as a "youth potion" (much superior to "bio-identical" hormones), which we then re-introduce back into our body at an older age. Still, we cannot escape the same result of an increased chance of growing cancerous cells. This is because we go against the laws of nature and ignore our body's biological clock that regulates and programs itself as a whole in a natural, graceful, and beautiful way.

How can we assist our bodies in making a comfortable and balanced transition during the natural aging process of the menopausal stage?

1) Emotional Self-Control: During the menopausal period, biological change is more of a yin deficiency in most women. There will be more heat, or yang activity, in the body and emotional changes due to the imbalance. When the heart organ is not balanced, there can be anxiety, panic attacks, heart palpitations, and sleeping pattern changes. If the liver organ is the main imbalance, there can be a quick temper, crying, impatience, and being easily stressed over things that were not stressors previously. Some women also feel depressed, fearful, and become suspicious. It is important to find ways to defuse anger, such as knowing when to walk away for a bit, use deep breathing, or find other ways to keep calm in order to avoid unnecessary confrontation. It can help to organize one's life and work schedule well, and to avoid trying to fulfill a long list of activities each day, but instead to give yourself more time to do things you find enjoyable and relaxing, keeping inner peace by whatever method works for you.

2. Lifestyle Modifications: To preserve and rejuvenate energy, be sure to have sufficient sleep, not over-exert yourself, and do moderate or gentle—not stressful—exercise, such as walking, hiking, Tai Chi, yoga, and Qigong.

3. TCM Food Therapy: The principle of the diet at this stage is to
    a) Nourish the spleen and the kidney organs;
    b) Consume nourishing yin food by eating more cooling foods, such as vegetables and fruits;
    c) Avoid hot and simulating foods such as alcohol, caffeinated drinks, pepper, and other hot spices that consume yin and lead

to more yang imbalance.

At the beginning of menopause, the spleen and kidneys start to show signs of deficiency. One aspect of spleen energy is to assist the body in controlling bleeding, or keeping the blood inside the blood vessels, without leakage. When this energy is deficient, there will be a heavier flow and continual bleeding from the uterus. Clinically, many middle-aged women (at the pre-menopausal stage) start to have heavy uterine bleeding. To prevent anemia at this stage, besides seeking proper treatment, women should consume more high-protein foods such as eggs, lean meat, dairy products, and more leafy green vegetables, tomatoes, peaches, and citrus fruits. When there is more heat and warmth in the body, and hypertension, one should consume more unprocessed whole grains, mushrooms, celery, apples, hawthorn fruit, green tea, sour dates, and mulberries to assist in lowering blood pressure, calming the heart, and helping with sleep. In order to strengthen kidney energy, one should consume more black-colored food, such as black beans, black sesame seeds, black rice, black fungus mushrooms, and walnuts.

The following are some diet therapies for women with a warm system during the menopausal period that I frequently recommend to patients in my clinic.

Morning Kidney-Nourishing Smoothie
Soy milk (room temperature)
One serving of super-green protein powder (soy-based protein)
Fresh blue/blackberries
Pine nuts
Two spoonfuls of non-fat yogurt

Blend all ingredients together to make approximately one 12-oz. serving.

Nourishing Yin Soup
Tofu: 200g, cut into big pieces
Lamb: 80g, cut into very thin pieces
Shrimp: 50g
Fresh ginger: 2 pieces
Salt

Put tofu and ginger in boiling water for ten minutes. Add lamb and shrimp, and cook for another 15-20 minutes. Add salt and other mild spices to taste, and serve.

4. Herbal Tea and Acupuncture Therapy: It is the philosophy of Chinese medicine to look at each individual as a whole entity; each individual has different degrees of disharmony within their own system. I strongly recommend that women in the menopausal period seek a TCM doctor for evaluation. The treatment plan will be customized to the individual according to the pattern diagnosis done by the TCM doctor. The doctor may formulate an individualized herbal formula to balance the body, provide food therapy recommendations, or suggest acupuncture, which is the best way to reduce stress and balance emotions. Most women see benefits after one or two acupuncture treatment sessions. For example, for a person with more kidney yin deficiency, the practitioner should use certain acupuncture points and herbs to nourish the kidney yin, and at the same time clear heat for balancing and eliminating the signs and symptoms related to yin deficiency. The selection of herbs and the dosage of each herb will depend on the degree of the body's disharmony, and most importantly, the experience of the Chinese herbalist.

Chapter 6
Food Therapy Modifications
According to Seasonal Changes

The natural environment provides vital conditions that humans and other life forms cannot live without. At the same time, a sudden or unusual change of environment can cause health problems. A Chinese proverb says that the relationship between human health and nature is like a boat on water: a boat needs water to float, but water can also destroy the boat. Similarly, TCM philosophy holds that humans and the universe are one. Food becomes part of the body after being consumed, but the four seasons (that is, environmental factors) are continually impacting the body externally.

We understand that environmental factors such as temperature, moisture, wind, seasons, and exposure to sunlight have a big impact on human physiological function. In fact, human physiology and metabolism are continually making changes in order to adjust to seasonal changes. In the spring, the weather gradually grows warmer, and the body starts to increase metabolism and consumption, while decreasing absorption of and the capacity to store nutrients. When the temperature decreases during winter, the body slows down its metabolism and increases absorption and storage, as animals do in hibernation. (For this reason, winter is the best time to take tonic herbs to strengthen the body and restore immunity.)

Besides the physiological changes that occur with seasonal change, humans tend to get different types of illnesses during different seasons. We tend to catch more colds and have headaches and nosebleeding in the spring; heat stroke and certain skin lesions in the summer; more gastritis and digestion problems in early fall; influenza and bronchitis during late fall; and more coughing, asthma, and respiratory tract infections in the winter season.

The principle of harmony between weather and food therapy may seem to contradict principles stated elsewhere, but the fact remains that food has a different impact on the body according to the season in which it is eaten. Chinese dietary philosophy suggests that you should embrace your native foods, in addition to eating locally grown, in-season foods. What is unhealthy about the modern diet is that many foods are now available all year long, being shipped from somewhere on the other side of the world, besides being chemically treated instead of grown naturally. Of course, homegrown and chemical-free products are the most nutritious and packed full of natural Qi.

Just as we need to adjust our clothing and dress more warmly in cooler seasons, or dress to maximize cooling in warmer seasons, so should we adjust our food choices according to seasonal changes.

Yang Sheng in the Springtime

The Characteristics of Life Forms in the Spring

Spring is the season of new birth and new growth as the weather begins to change from cold to warm. The mountain snows begin to melt, consuming some of the warmth from the air. Yang (warm) and yin (cold) energies start to interact as the yang energy rises, while the yin energy slowly retreats. The same process occurs inside the human body, as the yang energy rises to the surface and our skin pores open. This is why we are more sensitive to weather changes in the springtime, and can easily catch cold or may experience aches and pains related to the cold attacking our bodies when it is in a more vulnerable state with open pores. If we don't adapt to the changing climate in spring, we may become susceptible to seasonal health problems such as flu, pneumonia, or, in many cases, the recurrence of chronic disease. According to TCM, spring belongs to the wood element and dominates liver functioning. People should pay special attention to liver disharmony disorders.

Sleep Patterns in the Spring

Since spring is the season for sprouting and new growth throughout nature, and the human body follows the same natural law, more energy flows to the surface of the body, causing the body to naturally feel fatigued and need more sleep. There is a poem in Chinese history from the Tang dynasty: "Not knowing the high morning sun, in the spring sleeping until awakened by thousands of birds chatting." This is saying that in the springtime we need to sleep until late morning, even though we get to bed on time. It is important to adjust our sleep pattern to get additional rest, making sure all our body energy can rejuvenate and the yang energy can flow freely.

Diet Modification in the Spring

It is advisable to reduce the intake of sour flavors and increase sweet and mildly pungent flavors, as this facilitates the liver in regulating and free flow of Qi (vital energy) throughout the body. Examples of recommended foods for the spring include onions, leeks, leaf mustard, Chinese yams, wheat, dates, cilantro, mushrooms, spinach, and bamboo shoots. Fresh green and leafy vegetables should also be included in meals, and sprouts from seed are also valuable. In addition, uncooked, frozen, and fried foods should only be taken in moderation, since these are harmful to the spleen and stomach if consumed in large amounts. The cold winter keeps us indoors, consuming more meat and using more warm and hot spices. For this reason, people may develop a heat imbalance after winter, in the early spring, which leads to a dry throat, bad breath, constipation, a thick tongue coating, and yellowish urine. Foods like bananas, pears, water chestnuts, sugar cane, celery, and cucumber help to clear the excessive heat accumulated during winter.

The Principles of Choosing Food for the Spring Season
1. Choose more food with a sweet property: goji berries, barley, carrots, dates, coconuts, longan, mulberries, and melon.
2. Choose more food with a mild cooling property: soybeans, spinach, eggplant, bamboo, winter melon, cucumbers, mushrooms, tofu, celery, duck meat, duck eggs, liver, and multigrains.
3. Try to avoid too much pungent, hot and spicy, and deep-fried foods, because they will reinforce yang energy to an extreme, causing more sleep disorders, anxiety, dry throat, and skin disorders.
4. If one tends to have skin allergies, try to avoid shellfish, shrimp, and even fish, especially during the springtime.

Beneficial Foods for Springtime: Chicken, chicken liver, eggs, green vegetables, fresh fruit, tofu, and soybeans, which have a mild cooling property. Green tea is also recommended, alone or with white chrysanthemum flowers (3g); drink with honey.

Spring Dishes for Food Therapy

Chrysanthemum Chicken

Chicken meat: 250g, cut into small pieces
Fresh chrysanthemum flower petals: 30g, rinsed clean
Green onion: one, cut into small pieces
Ginger: 5g, cut into small pieces
Cooking wine: one tbsp
Tapioca starch: one tsp, dissolved in water
Salt
Egg white from one egg

Mix cut-up chicken together with the salt, cooking wine, ginger, green onion, and egg white. After warming oil in a frying pan, add the chicken and stir while cooking until done. Then add the tapioca starch, stirring until smooth. Last, add the chrysanthemum flower petals, stirring a couple of times, and serve.

Function: Strengthens the spleen and nourishes Qi, nourishes the liver, benefits the eyes, and calms the heart and spirit.

Spinach Rice Soup
Spinach: 250g, rinsed and cut into small pieces
Spring rice (or sushi rice): 250g
Salt

Cook rice with water to make a soup, cooking until the rice is soft and smooth, and then add in the spinach, with salt or other spices, cooking until soft. Serve along with meal twice a week.

Function: Nourishes blood and Qi, moistens the large intestines, helping with constipation, and assists with blood pressure control.

Nourishing the Spirit and Emotions during the Spring

Springtime is "wood element" season, coordinated with liver organ energy. As we know from the previous chapter, the liver organ likes to have free-flowing energy and not be stagnant. Otherwise, one becomes easily angered, irritable, and depressed. Daoist and Yang Sheng experts in TCM history tell us that in the springtime, one should not attempt to kill any forms of life on earth; one should not attempt to make economic or other types of gain (since desire drains energy from the heart and causes liver stagnation); and one should not punish or criticize others, but appreciate them. One should enjoy and appreciate the springtime for bringing new yang life or positive energy to earth. Hike in the wilderness to see the wildflowers; listen to the birds singing; and bathe in the spring sunshine and breezes. One should sing and dance near water, appreciating spring's nourishment of spirit and soul.

Yang Sheng in Summertime

The Characteristics of Life Forms in the Summer

In the summer, there is more sunlight, bringing life to nature; there is more yang energy that makes the plants grow faster by absorbing energy from the heavenly summer sun (photosynthesis). People are more active and energetic, and the body's Qi and blood become relatively more vigorous and more toward the surface of the body than during the other seasons. With all the yang activity and the warm environment, the body needs to sweat in order to balance its temperature. We should encourage the body to sweat in a balanced way, not excessively. The sweating process and all the yang activity consume the body's energy, which is why we naturally lose weight during the summer. If we always stay in air-conditioned rooms during the summer, the body has no chance to sweat, discharge dampness, and consume some of the accumulated body weight carried over from winter. In this case, the body tends to retain dampness and phlegm, with energy stagnation and weight gain.

Sleep Patterns in the Summer

Summer season is naturally the strongest yang (sun and daylight) season—with corresponding weakness of yin (night) energy in the universe—and the human body follows the same natural laws accordingly. That is why we tend to go to sleep late and wake up early in our natural summer sleep pattern, which fits with the more-yang, less-yin summer season. The body energy is consumed more in the summer because of less sleep during the night. This is why, in many cultures, it is customary to have a midday nap break during the hot summer. This custom not only avoids the hottest time of the day, preventing heat stroke, but more importantly, it provides the body with the needed extra sleep time that is lost during the summer nights. It is a logical custom, and in fact, enhances work performance.

Diet Modification in the Summer

TCM teaches that the physiological changes that take place during the seasonal change to summer make the heart over-work, and there is too much yang-Qi flowing outward to the exterior part of the body. According to the five-element theory, an over-functioning heart restricts the functioning of the lungs. It is advisable to eat more food with pungent flavors, which helps the lung Qi, and to reduce bitter flavors (bitter-tasting food drains the heart). This enhances the lungs and maintains the normal sweating mechanism in the summer. Sweat is the fluid of the heart; excessive sweating scatters heart-Qi and weakens the mind, causing symptoms like being easily annoyed and restless, and having low spirits and sleeping difficulties. Foods with sour and salty flavors help to ease these symptoms. Summer is hot; if there is rain, it will be hot and humid. The heat forces the body's pores to open and to sweat. The process of sweating causes the body to lose fluid (nutritive fluid) and consumes body energy. This is why summer is the most energy-consuming season and disturbs the fluid and electrolyte balance of the body, leading to lethargy, weakness, fever, thirst, lack of appetite, and possibly loose bowels.

Some foods are recommended for keeping the body cool and balanced, such as bitter melon, watermelon, strawberries, tomatoes, mung beans, cucumbers, wax gourd, lotus root, lotus seeds, Job's tears, bean sprouts, duck, and fish. In general, the daily diet should contain more vegetables and fruit at this time in order to stimulate the appetite and provide adequate fluids. Warm and cooked foods ensure that the digestive system works more effectively; too many greasy, raw, and frozen foods can damage the digestive system and lead to poor appetite, diarrhea, or stomach upset. It is a Chinese tradition in summer to make soups for clearing summer heat, eliminating dampness, and promoting digestion.

Ginger for the Summer

There is a Chinese saying: "Summer ginger and winter turnip." In the summer, we tend to eat fruit and other cold, raw foods due to the hot weather and the availability of fresh fruits and vegetables; however, these foods tend to compromise the digestive system. This is why in the summer, more ginger is added to the diet, in order to warm and harmonize the digestive system, balancing the summer diet.

The Principles of Choosing Food in the Summer Season

1. To clear heat and expel dampness and toxins from the body, one can drink mint tea, *pei lan ye* (*Eupatorium fortunei herba*) or *huo xiang ye* (patchouli or *Agastache* plant), 10g each, with 30g charred *mai ya* (barley sprout), and 3g *gan cao* (licorice root). Make a concoction to make tea.
2. To clear heat, drain dampness, and generate fluid in the body to stop thirst, drink watermelon juice, mung bean soup, and lightly salted water, if dehydrated.
3. To nourish the spleen and stomach, strengthen Qi, and rejuvenate yin, drink *Astragalus* tea, or American ginseng tea if extremely fatigued, even after clearing heat and sufficient hydration.
4. Avoid pungent, dry, and sour food, as well as deep-fried food.

Nourishing the Spirit and the Emotions during the Summer

The summer season corresponds to the element of fire, which is related to the characteristic of the heart organ. In the summer, heat can exhaust the body and weaken the heart energy, leading to irritability, a short temper, heart palpitations, and a loss of mental concentration. The best way to nourish the spirit is to keep an inner calm and mentally cool down the body with meditation, emptying the mind and not reacting to external stimuli. There is a saying in Chinese: "A cooling sensation follows the calming of the heart."

Preventing Winter Disease during the Summer

Chronic diseases that often recur in the winter are related to kidney and lung energy deficiency, such as chronic bronchitis, emphysema, asthma, chronic arthritis, and chronic diarrhea. For example, chronic bronchitis in the elderly often recurs during the winter. Summer is the best time for these patients to begin treating and nourishing kidney energy by taking nourishing kidney yang herbs for a month, or putting herbal patches on acu-points on related organ meridians for three months. This proves to be very effective in preventing recurrence during the winter season. The same applies for the yang child with asthma; during the summer, treat for three months with an herbal patch. For most children, consistent treatment for three summers increases immunity, eliminates hypersensitivity, and stops chronic childhood asthma.

Yang Sheng in the Fall

The Characteristics of Life Forms in the Fall

The weather changes gradually from hot to cool, with yang energy starting to go inward and growing weaker, and yin energy growing stronger. Fall is the season of yang and yin exchange and transformation. At the same time, most life forms start to mature, ripen, and fall in the autumn. TCM teaches that autumn correlates with the lung organs, which dominate the skin, respiration, body fluid metabolism, blood circulation, immunity, and the emotion of melancholy. Since the vigorous summer is over, in the body, everything needs to turn inward to prepare for the harsh winter. The Yang Sheng principle in the fall season is "consolidate."

Sleep Patterns in the Fall

Since yang energy starts to go from outer in summer, to inward in the fall, the body naturally adjusts its sleep time accordingly. *Inner Classic* states, "Our body goes to sleep and wakes up early, like the rooster, during the three months of the fall season." Sleeping early in the fall season is just following the natural way of yang energy going inward, and rising early with the early sunrise, and still having more yang energy from the sun. Getting up early in the morning is better for moving the lung energy smoothly outward to prevent too much inward movement of energy.

During the fall, the weather can change dramatically from the residual heat of the summer to cool down at night. There may be four seasonal changes in one day, or four seasonal changes within a ten-mile radius. It is important to dress properly, according to temperature changes.

Nourishing the Spirit and Emotions during the Fall

Fall, with its cool, dry air, is the best season for traveling and enjoying the beauty of nature. However, with the weather cooling down and the temperature falling, with leaves turning yellow and falling, and plants and flowers starting to wither, some experience a sense of sadness and melancholy, especially those with weak lung energy, which is the body's defensive energy. These people tend to have depression or irritability and may undergo emotional changes during this season. In order to nourish good spirits, *Inner Classic* recommends, "During the fall season, one should keep optimism, inner tranquility, and a calm spirit, constrain overreacting, and avoid outer negativity."

In Chinese culture, there is a centuries-old fall holiday on September 9th on the lunar calendar. Since the number 9 is a yang number, the holiday is called Double Yang Day. Traditionally, besides celebrating the holiday with friends and family, one should also go hiking and enjoy the view from high places. There is also a moon festival during this season. These holidays provide more opportunities to gather together socially and to feel happy, nourishing the spirit. This is the same in many Western cultures, when there are many holidays during the fall season. Thanksgiving, for example, is a great tradition, when everyone wants to be with family and friends for a cultural celebration, emotional bonding, and nurturing the spirit. One way to keep up good spirits during the fall and winter season is to socialize more with friends and family. Many cultures have more holidays during the second half of the year, providing the opportunity for togetherness and bonding.

Diet Modification in the Fall

Choice of food is important to ensure that the body adjusts to the changing seasons. The dry weather usually causes an itchy throat, a dry nose, chapped lips, rough skin, hair loss, and dry stools. Add more food to the diet that can promote the production of body fluids and a lubricating effect throughout the body. Beneficial foods for this dry season include lily bulbs, white fungus, nuts and seeds, pears, lotus roots, pumpkin, black sesame seeds, sweet rice, pineapples, honey, soy milk, and dairy products. It is advisable to eat more food with sour flavors, such as pineapple, apple, grapefruit, and lemon, and reduce pungent flavors, such as onions, ginger, and peppers. Sour foods have astringent properties, preventing the loss of body fluids, while pungent foods induce perspiration. The body needs extra fluids to counteract the dry environment, which is why it is a Chinese tradition to eat porridge (congee) for breakfast and soup for dinner that is made with the above ingredients.

The Principles of Choosing Food in the Fall Season

1. Eat less greasy and baked/barbecued food.
2. Avoid pungent and hot, spicy food in order to preserve more body fluids.
3. Eat more nourishing fluid and moisturizing food, as mentioned above.

Preventing Disease during the Fall Season

In the fall, there is a tendency to suffer from digestive system disorders, such as enterogastritis, diarrhea, dysentery, and dryness. Try to avoid too much unclean, cold, and raw food during this season. One can take herbs, such as *ban lan gen* (*Isatis* root) and *ma chi xian* tea (pursiane) to prevent gastrointestinal infection.

If the fall season is dry, it can cause lip, nasal, and throat dryness; dry skin; and constipation. Chinese herbs that nourish yin and fluid production and protect the lungs are American ginseng, *sha shen* (*Glehnia* root), apricot kernels, lily bulbs, and *chuan bei mu* (*Fritillaria cirrhosa bulbus*).

Yang Sheng in Wintertime

The Characteristics of Life Forms in Winter

In winter, living things slow down to save energy, while some animals hibernate. Winter season is yin season, cold, and related to the kidneys. During the winter, yin energy is at its peak, while yang energy is submerged. All the plants are withered, while the human body's activity, or metabolism, is slow and at a relatively low level. It is also the season when humans conserve energy, build strength, and store more yin energy (materials) in the body, while spending less Qi (yang activity). This is the best season for taking supplements that coordinate the natural winter seasonal activity of rebuilding, restoring, and rejuvenating the body and the organs as a prelude in preparation for spring. So the characteristic of winter is "restoration and conservation."

Cold winter not only brings cold winds, but, in some areas, dampness. The cold and dampness together can cause many health problems and some cold and kidney deficiency-related diseases recurrent during the winter season.

Dress appropriately. If one dresses too warm during the winter, it will disturb yang, and the yang energy will go to the skin surface, opening the pores rather than remaining submerged. Then the cold pathogens can easily invade the body. If one dresses too lightly, the cold temperature will consume more of the body's yang energy, leading to weakening of the body's defensive energy, with the tendency to catch cold and have allergies. *Inner Classic* states: "During the winter season, one should preserve the body's essence by restraining their sexuality for preventing disease in the coming spring." This is an important Yang Sheng method for conserving and strengthening the body and kidney essence during the winter, to prevent diseases that are common during early spring. As we know, animals refrain from sexual activity and preserve their body energy during the winter season, and are ready to mate in early spring for healthier offspring. Humans, as part of nature, do the same.

Sleep Patterns in the Winter

During the winter, the daytime is short, yang-time is weak, and yin-time is high. The same goes for the human body, with the yang energy at its lowest, thus requiring more sleep naturally during the winter. We should sleep early and get up late, going to work after sunrise.

Nourishing the Spirit and Emotions during the Winter

In the winter, yang energy is naturally deep inside. In order not to disturb the yang energy, one should keep the emotions even and refrain from too much desire to conserve the body's energy and be prepared for the coming spring.

Diet Modification in the Winter

TCM teaches that our diet should be adapted to focus on enriching yin and subduing yang, which means we should consume appropriate fats and high-protein foods. Mutton, beef, goose, duck, eggs, rabbit meat, Chinese yams, sesame seeds, glutinous rice, dates, longan, black fungus, bamboo shoots, mushrooms, leeks, and nuts are common ingredients in Chinese dishes at this time. Winter corresponds to the organ of kidney according to the five elements theory; hyperactive kidneys inhibit the heart, which leads to palpitations, cardiac pain, limb coldness, and fatigue. It is advisable to eat more food with bitter flavors, while reducing salty flavors, so as to promote a healthy heart and reduce the workload of the kidneys. Foods with bitter flavors include apricots, asparagus, celery, coffee, tea, grapefruit, hops, kohlrabi, lettuce, radish leaves, kale, vinegar, and wine.

Some people may eat too many hot pots or high-calorie foods, causing excessive heat to accumulate in the lungs and stomach. They may experience problems such as bronchitis, sore throat, peptic ulcer, and skin problems; thus it is necessary to balance the diet with a certain amount of cool-property vegetables, as well as water. Remember the Chinese saying, "Summer ginger and winter turnip." Turnips are cold-property vegetables. During the winter, we tend to eat more warm food, with warm spices, using turnips to make a soup to balance the warmth and soothe the digestive system, as well as clearing extra heat.

Winter is also a good time to boost the natural constitution of the body and improve symptoms associated with chronic conditions. Since a person's appetite tends to increase in the winter when the body's metabolism is lower, the nutrients absorbed from food can be stored more easily. Energizing herbs, such as ginseng, wolfberries (goji berries), *Angelica*, *Rehmannia* root, *Astragalus*, and medicinal mushrooms can be used for this purpose. It is a trend for Chinese restaurants to prepare various medicinal courses, choosing these ingredients in the winter season to strengthen the kidneys.

Watch salt intake carefully during the winter. During the cold days of winter, the body has less yang on its surface, so the skin pores are closed, and there is less perspiration. Along with limiting salt intake, eat foods with a bitter taste, which will help maintain the balance between the kidneys and the heart.

Disease Prevention in the Winter Season

Winter is the best season of the year to take supplements and use TCM food therapy to restore, strengthen, and rejuvenate body. To achieve this, one can take tonic herbs and/or use food therapy, with the latter being the best choice. (To apply food therapy according to age and body constitution, refer to Chapters 5 and 7).

Besides taking proper nutrition, moderate exercise is very important during this season to increase Qi and blood circulation, and to bring more defensive Qi to the body's surface to protect it from pathogens. There is an old folk saying in Chinese: "Move in the winter to avoid disease; a lazy day in winter will end by taking a concoction."

Dress properly to avoid extreme cold that can trigger cardiovascular diseases, such as heart attack and stroke, as well as cold- and damp-related diseases, such as chronic bronchitis, asthma, and arthritic pain.

Chapter 7
Food Therapy According to Different Types of Body Constitutions

We often notice how certain people always feel warm and clammy, while others feel cold all time. Some people have weak digestive systems, and when under stress, some tend to have diarrhea, and others constipation. Certain people have very nice skin that is shiny, with few wrinkles and spots, while others have large pores, oily skin, and acne. Some people have beautiful, thick, shiny hair, and others have thin, soft, and weak hair that becomes grey prematurely. Certain people are prone to an emotional response of sadness and worry, while others quickly overreact with aggression. We also note that some people rarely get sick, and when they do, they recover quickly, without many complications; others seem to get sick rather easily and take longer to get well. All these individual differences—the response to environmental changes, the emotional tendencies, the kinds of illnesses typical to an individual, and the body's response to certain diets—all depend on the individual's "body constitution."

What is body constitution?

Body constitution is a relative consistency of body structure with the intrinsic being of the body—the personality and psychological dynamic constituted from the intrinsic being or genetic factors, and the lifestyle, diet, living conditions, and social environment after birth. In fact, a simple description of body constitution is an individual's Jing, Qi, and Shen (Three Treasures) manifesting as a whole.

The Importance of Understanding our Body's Constitution

If we know our individual body constitution at an early age, we can modify our lifestyle to prevent certain diseases after we reach adulthood.

We can follow a diet and exercise regimen that is good and appropriate for our type of constitution. For example, during the hot summer, some people feel refreshed after eating cold, fresh fruit, while others get diarrhea after eating cold or raw foods like fruit or salad. Some people love to eat hot and spicy food and feel that the body loosens up and feels lighter afterward. Others, however, will break out in pimples, blisters, or rashes and suffer from heartburn as a result.

If we know our body constitution, we know the emotional response we tend to have. It is then possible to find the remedy for balancing the body and the emotional response. We will also know what kind of climate best suits us.

If we know our body constitution, we will recognize when our body becomes unbalanced, and it will signal us to be proactive in preventing illness. If we are balanced, we will be pain-free, even-tempered, and energetic. Once we begin to develop allergies to things we had no previous problems with, we begin to feel more pain in the body and have sleep and digestion issues, as well as being more emotionally sensitive, even though all blood tests, x-rays, MRIs, etc. are normal. This indicates that our body's "balanced status" has tilted to a "sub-clinical condition," "the third condition," or, as I like to call it, the "sub-healthy status."

Once our body has reached "sub-healthy status," we should be more proactive in modifying our diet and lifestyle in order to restore our body to a healthy balance and prevent disease. If we do not understand our body constitution, we might just do the opposite. For example, several years ago, I had a patient who had been suffering from diarrhea resulting from colitis for about two years. The stool was watery and sometimes contained undigested food particles. She felt cold and had a tendency to gain weight. Her body constitution was colder, with low energy (low yang energy) in the digestive system—thus her inability to digest food. However, someone had suggested to her that she should detoxify her body with a raw food diet to cure her disease. She took the advice, staying with it for more than a year, with the result that her body only felt colder and her diarrhea did not stop. Instead, it grew worse, with incidents of diarrhea over ten times per day at times. She gained a lot of weight, had dry skin, lost hair, and was fatigued all the time. The cold, raw food only exacerbated the patient's cold and yang energy deficient condition.

Body constitution is the answer to why one form of diet, one form of exercise, one form of therapy, or even one supplement cannot fit everyone and cannot be the answer for every problem. I do not agree with the common practice in our society of trying to convince people that a single mystery therapy, supplement, or modality is appropriate for every individual and every condition.

Can the body constitution be changed?

Yes, certain body constitutions can be changed, but to a limited extent. First of all, it is very rare that an individual exhibits only one body constitution. Usually, an individual exhibits more than one body constitution type, but one predominates over another at different times of life. The predominant constitution can be changed during different stages of life by aging, lifestyle, and changes in one's living environment and conditions.

Body constitution can change after years of lifestyle modification or chronic disease, by adding one type of constitution or change to another. For example, a woman who predominantly felt cold during early age, upon reaching middle age, after multiple childbirths and years of excessive tobacco and alcohol consumption, will find her body now feels predominantly warm, with dry skin, dry throat, and fragile bones. In this example, the body constitution changed from yang deficiency to yin deficiency.

Body Constitution from Parental Inheritance

This part of the body constitution cannot be changed, such as the family tendency to form certain kinds of tumors or to develop diabetes or heart disease. But this does not mean that a person who is born with a certain body constitution cannot do anything about it.

The body's constitution is also relatively consistent with lifestyle, diet, social conditions, and environment. In this regard, constitution can be changed to a limited extent over the long term by modifying lifestyle and diet, and by changing the climate in which one lives, as well as the living conditions.

In Chinese culture, most people understand the old saying: "To recover from disease, only one-third needs to be treated; the other two-thirds needs Tiao Yang." In narrow terms relating only to the healing process, *Tiao Yang* means to convalesce through care, rest, and nourishment to promote longevity and reach maximum life span. Tiao Yang is both a physical and emotional practice that consists of adjusting lifestyle, diet, and spiritual practice according to one's stage of life, body constitution, environmental changes, and current health condition.

How to achieve Tiao Yang and modify the diet to restore health? One must understand one's constitution and Tiao Yang accordingly.

The Eight Types of Body Constitution and How Each Manifests According to Traditional Chinese Medicine

There are eight types of body constitutions. Within each individual, there may be more than one type together, but one or two types will predominate.

1. Ping Heng Type (Balanced type)
2. Yang Xu Type (Yang deficiency type)
3. Yin Xu Type (Yin deficiency type)
4. Qi Xu Type (Qi or Energy deficiency type)

5. Xue Xu Type (Blood deficiency type)
6. Qi Yu Type (Qi or Energy stagnation type)
7. Xue Yu Type (Blood stagnation type)
8. Tan Shi Type (Dampness and Phlegm type)

1) Ping Heng Type: Balanced

There is a small percentage of the population living in the city that has this type of body constitution. These types of people are physically and emotionally balanced. They live longer and are emotionally more stable, with a more positive personality. They are more open-minded, flexible, non-confrontational, generous, and more satisfied and happy overall. They rarely get sick, and suffer less physical pain and insomnia in old age. Their bodies have greater adaptability to environmental changes than most people.

Characteristics of a Balanced Individual
This includes two parts:
   I. Physical Well-Being
- Good spirit in the eye
- Normal breathing rhythm
- Regular urination and bowel movements
- Non-rapid, strong, regular pulse
- Balanced physical figure/physique
- Healthy facial complexion
- Healthy, strong, natural teeth
- Sharp hearing
- Flexibility of the back and legs, without pain
- A clear voice
- Shiny and normal hair color
- Normal appetite

   II. Psychological and Spiritual Well-Being
- Happy and satisfied

- Good memory

There are several places in the world where people live longer than the rest of the world. Most long-lived people live simple, beautiful, natural lives with a great deal of satisfaction and happiness. There is a county in the southern part of China, Ba Ma Xian, in the mountainous area of Gui Zhou Province. On average, the people who live there are over 90 years old. Ba Ma is a beautiful, rural county with rivers and mountains. The villagers live together with several generations, eating local food of mostly rice, corn, yams, and vegetables. The most striking characteristic of those who live long is a life of simplicity and happiness.

<u>Maintaining Balance through Lifestyle</u>

You are very lucky if you have this type of body constitution, and it is important to maintain it by not doing anything unnatural, such as ingesting man-made supplements. One should get all of one's nutrition from seasonal, regional, organic foods. Constant movement should arise from walking, swimming, Tai Chi, and meditation—all in moderation, so as not to force the body to perform or simply to build big muscles for show. Inner peace is one of the most important factors in this group of people. The more desire, the more vanity, the more pretention one has, the more disappointment, the more dissatisfaction, the more unhappiness one feels in the end, as one's energy is exhausted and eroding emotions shorten one's life.

2) Yang Xu Type: Yang Deficiency

Yang energy is warm, moving, activating energy with a lot of vitality. Manifestation of organ function and an individual's vitality depend on the yang energy. Of course, the yang energy depends on yin substance (body's essence, blood, fluid, and nutrition) to rejoice. In other words, the yang energy manifests that there is a yin substance in the body to support it, like the fire and the wood. The fire as yang energy depends on the existing wood, and the continuing fire depends on the wood substance, the tangible form of energy within the wood. In our body, the original yang energy comes from the kidney essence, the source of yin energy within the kidneys.

Characteristics of the Yang Deficiency Type

This individual tends to feel colder than other people, with cold limbs, pale complexion, fatigue, and no desire to speak. They may feel coldness in the upper abdomen, a tingling sensation, more saliva, or long and clear urination. If there is yang deficiency in the heart, a person often has a sensation of pressure and pain in the chest that can radiate to the upper back muscle. If there is yang deficiency that impacts digestion or the spleen, one tends to have watery diarrhea with non-digested food particles, and water retention in the lower legs. There is also a type of diarrhea that is caused by kidney yang deficiency. This type if diarrhea occurs upon waking in the morning, or when just awakening from sleep. Besides this type of diarrhea, a kidney yang deficient person tends to have frequent urination at night, and cold pain above the knees and elbows. Men with kidney yang deficiency tend to have lower sexual desire, erectile dysfunction, premature ejaculation, and an inability to perform. Women might have menstrual delay, a history of miscarriage, and other infertility issues if the yang energy deficiency is not corrected and balanced by lifestyle changes.

Since the kidney yang energy is the original yang energy in the body, it controls our bone structure and longevity. The yang deficiency body constitution tends to have osteoporosis. This is why TCM uses nourishing yang herbs and a diet that treats and prevents osteoporosis.

People with yang deficiency not only tend to have diarrhea and a feeling of coldness; they also tend to gain weight. This type of weight gain is from the body's tendency to retain water, since the body has no strength or yang energy to transform water and food.

In the clinic, we see many people with colitis fall into yang deficiency. It is not simply a matter of stopping the diarrhea, or using immune suppressor drugs—which continue to suppress the body's yang energy—to treat the diarrhea symptom only. I have already mentioned my patient who suffered from chronic diarrhea due to colitis. After failing to improve through the use of steroids and other immune suppressor medications, she had taken the advice of a friend to join the Raw Food Society to detoxify her body. She initially came to my office for shoulder joint pain treatment only. Her facial complexion was very pale; she had coldness in the limbs, with dry, scaly skin and very thin, dry hair. Her body type was slightly overweight. After treating her shoulder pain, we discovered that she had had an accident on the treatment bed, but with only liquid feces and no stool substance. She then told me her history with colitis and all that she had gone through, including her raw food diet.

In the culture of the West, most people still are not aware of how much Traditional Chinese Medicine can do. Westerners believe that TCM consists only of acupuncture, and that it treats only pain. However, before this patient left, I advised her on how to prepare a special congee (porridge) diet therapy with warm, cooked, soft, bland ingredients, to be eaten until the following week, when I would re-evaluate her condition. A week later, just before her appointment, the patient called me. She was very excited that her symptoms and frequency of diarrhea had already improved 50% just by modifying her diet! I do not mention this case to cast aspersions on any medication therapy or raw food diet therapy. My only intention is to point out that it is important to determine whether any good treatment or therapy fits our body constitution, and to stress that there is no one blanket therapy for everyone.

If an adult had a history of asthma as an infant, they will sometimes tell you that they were born with asthma, or experienced some kind of developmental delay during childhood. This indicates that this person may have had yang (kidney) energy deficiency since birth.

Their body constitution is the yang (kidney) deficiency type. This type of body constitution requires lifestyle changes and an appropriate diet to balance this deficiency, in order to avoid many physical illnesses upon reaching adulthood. Sometimes we see a family take their young child to see a TCM doctor to evaluate their child's body constitution and get advice for an appropriate diet for the child, in order to prevent sickness and ensure better health in adulthood.

We can see that people with depleted kidney yang energy tend to manifest later in life with premature aging; bone structure problems, including teeth, hair, and hearing problems at a young age; fertility and sexuality problems; and early menopausal and immunity disorders that may lead to many other physical disorders and the formation of tumors.

The emotional state of someone with this constitution type tends to be inward, with feelings of fear, low self-esteem, and depression.

Causes of Yang Deficiency
  a) Lifestyle has a significant impact on this type of body constitution. Many professional athletes who engage in competitive sports and workers who perform hard, physical labor tend to exhaust the body's Qi (energy), which later on compromises the yang, with lumbar and joint pain and bone structure problems.
  b) Long-term consumption of food that has cold properties can damage the body's yang.
  c) A common practice in our society is the abuse of certain supplements and laxatives by taking them without knowing whether they are a fit for one's body constitution, as well as self-detoxification through the use of purgative and harsh supplements that damage the spleen Qi and yang energy.
  d) Chemotherapy treatment and the taking of certain medications, especially the long-term abuse of antibiotics and steroids that exhaust the spleen Qi and yang, which result in retaining

phlegm in the body. We can see that the patient has extreme Qi and yang deficiency so that the body loses its immunity defense, as well as decreased production of Qi and blood, hair loss, end of bone (teeth) loss, and loss of normal strength (energy).

e) Some individuals' body constitution changes to yang deficiency after suffering a chronic disease.

Tiao Yang Methods for the Yang Deficiency Type

Temperate Climate: For the yang deficiency type, it is important to choose a suitable living environment. This type cannot tolerate cold weather or a cold winter season, and must dress warmly in order to avoid many health problems, both acute and chronic. In order to increase cold tolerance during the wintertime, the yang deficiency type should strengthen and nourish yang energy during the summertime. A simple way to do this is to sunbathe 20-30 times during the summer, for 20-30 minutes per sunbath.

Sleep Climate: The yang deficient person should not sleep with the air-conditioning on or out-of-doors in the summertime. In summer, the yang energy comes to the body's surface; the pores of the skin are open, and the muscles and tendons of the body are more relaxed. Thus, the cooler air from air-conditioning, and the outdoor night air, can damage the body's yang energy. This is why people who suffer from Bell's palsy, numbness of the peripheral limbs, or circulation issues are more prone to experience problems during the summer season.

Sleep Schedule: We should understand that nighttime is the body's yin time—compared with yang time, which is in the daytime. This means the body needs rest, rejuvenation, and replenishment at night. During the yin-time (nighttime), the body's yin generates more yin material, such as blood, for more yang activity during the daytime.

The body's performance, or yang activity, is a manifestation of yin substance in the body. In the daytime (yang-time), the body's Qi and yang energy go to the surface in order for the body to perform. This is our body's natural biological clock. In bio-medicine, we see the same pattern of our body's natural hormones from the adrenal glands. In the early morning, adrenal gland hormones gradually increase; they start to decrease in the early afternoon, along with the body's metabolic rate and basic body temperature. A long-term night-shift worker's schedule goes completely contrary to the body's biological clock, and in the end will exhaust the body's yin substance, showing yin deficiency first and totally depleting yang in the long term.

It is recommended that you follow the body's biological clock and go to sleep early at night, before 10:30 p.m., to restore the body's energy.

Balancing the Emotions: The yang deficiency type is often introverted, with suppressed emotions or "inward emotions," and with "downward emotions," such as fear, sadness, and to some degree, depression. Maintaining a good connection with family, friends, and other sources of ongoing emotional support can be very important for the well-being of this type.

Physical Exertion: Workers in certain professions tend to suffer yang deficiency at a relatively young age, including professional athletes, hard physical laborers, and long-term night-shift workers. These professions force the body to perform without giving it enough time to rejuvenate itself. It may only be impacting the body on a superficial level, or the Qi level, and at this level, the body can easily recover simply by resting and sleeping more. However, most young people in these professions tend to ignore their body's need for rest, preferring to push the body to perform beyond its limits. For a long period of time, or later on in life, the Qi level depletion will impact on a deeper level, at the expense of the body's essence, which leads to yang deficiency of the kidneys. This is especially the case with those who take stimulants to force the body to perform.

Exercise: Exercises for the yang deficiency person include Qigong therapy and kidney Qi, also called Yuan Qi (the original Qi). The practice of Qigong nourishes kidney Qi.

Diet: This type should avoid food and drink that has cold properties and cold temperatures. It is common for people to eat cold salads and fruits, such as watermelon, and to drink cold drinks in the summertime when it is hot. While it is refreshing for most people, for the person who is yang deficient, there will be repercussions later in the year, after the summer season. For some, there will be instantaneous results from eating too much cold, raw food. These symptoms can include loose stools and diarrhea, as well as weight gain, which is why some people are prone to gain weight in the hot summer after consuming too much cold food.

Remember the old Chinese saying, "Winter turnip and summer ginger." This means you need more ginger in the summer, rather than a lot of cold fruit. With warm, spicy ginger, you will have better digestion and ensure a healthier digestive system. By adding more ginger to your diet in the summer, you can counteract the consumption of cold food and drink during the warm season. If you go south to Mexico, during the summer along the street, it is very interesting to see that local farmers will serve you fresh fruit by adding a pinch of hot pepper powder on top of the fruit.

Other: For this type, it is also important to avoid taking excessive laxatives, colon therapy treatment, and any harsh detoxification therapy that can damage the body's yang. It is also important to avoid engaging in sexual activity at a young age, or excessive sexual activity at any age; as well as having multiple childbirths in close succession, or multiple abortions or miscarriages—all of which are the biggest contributors to the consumption of kidney essence and exhaustion of the body's yang energy.

TCM Food Therapy for Yang Deficiency

Foods that suit yang deficiency include spring rice, sweet rice, millet, barley, yam, potatoes, Chinese red dates, carrots, shitake mushrooms, organic chicken, deer meat, organic beef, and lamb.

The best seasons to nourish yang are spring and summer. During the summer season, I recommend more soups with meat and herbs.

Cong Rong Chicken

Organic chicken meat: 250g, cut into small pieces
Rou cong rong (broomrape): 30g, boiled in water to extract the concentrated herbal juice
Fresh chestnuts: 15 pieces, shells removed
Yi yi ren (coix seeds): 15g
Shiitake mushrooms: 5 pieces, pre-soaked to soften, then cut into small pieces.)
Fresh ginger, green onion, and salt

Stir-fry the chicken meat in a frying pan, then add the fresh ginger and green onion together. Add the *rou cong rong* (broomrape, fleshy stem) herbal juice, and the rest of the ingredients. Boil until well done. Serve as a dish with your regular meal.

Function: Strengthens the kidneys and yang; consolidates essence. For fatigue, cold limbs with lower sexual desire, and performance consistent with kidney yang deficiency.

Clove (Ding Xiang) Duck

Half of a whole duck.
Ding xiang (clover flower buds): 3g

Rou gui (cinnamon - inner bark): 3g
Rou dou kou (nutmeg seeds): 5g
Ginger, green onion, cumin, salt, cooking wine, and a small amount of dark brown sugar

Boil the clover, cinnamon, and nutmeg together in water for 20 minutes, then pour off the herbal juice. Repeat again by adding more water to boil the three herbs again for another 20 minutes, making a second juice extract. Combine the two juice extracts together to make approximately half a gallon. Use the herbal juice to boil the duck, adding the rest of the ingredients, to taste. Spoon the herbal juice over the duck as it boils, until the duck turns a dark red color and is well done. Serve as a dish with your meal.

Function: Warms and strengthens the stomach and spleen. Helps to dry dampness. For treatment of diarrhea and abdominal pain due to coldness.

Fresh Shrimp Soup
Fresh live shrimp: 100g
Astragalus: 30g, boiled in water for 25 minutes at a low temperature to get the herbal extract
Ginger, salt, cooking wine

Use the herbal juice to boil the shrimp with the other ingredients for 10 minutes.

Serve once a week; eat the shrimp and drink the soup broth.

Function: Warms the abdomen and limbs; strengthens energy and body immunity.

Wild Yam Lamb

Organic lamb meat: 250g, cut into 4 x 2 cm and mixed well with
 salt, fresh ginger, cooking wine, and starch/flour
Fresh wild Chinese yams: 100g, cut into thin pieces
Black fungal mushrooms: 30g, soaked in water until they
 expand, then washed and torn into small pieces
Fresh ginger and green onions, cut into small pieces

Stir-fry the lamb meat with oil until done. Remove meat from the pan and set aside. Add fresh ginger and onions to the hot pan, using the leftover oil, and brown. Add wild yams and mushrooms, with salt and cooking wine, until the yam changes color. Add the cooked lamb and stir together. Finally, add a little more starch to make everything smooth. Serve as a dish with your meal.

Function: Nourishes yang energy, nourishes blood, and warms kidneys to treat fatigue, dizziness, and weakness of the lumbar and the knees.

TCM Herbal Therapy for Yang Deficiency

There are many Chinese herbs for warming yang and nourishing the kidneys, liver, and heart. However, a professional is needed to recommend the proper herbal therapy. Commonly used yang tonic herbs include deer antlers, gecko, *Cordyceps* fungi, wild walnuts, cinnamon, *ba ji tain* (*Morinda* root), *bu gu zhi* (*Psoralea* fruit), *tu si zi* (*Cuscuta* seeds) and *yin yang hou* (*Epimedium*, aerial parts). These herbs can be integrated into TCM food therapy.

3) Yin Xu Type: Yin Deficiency

Yin is water, cool, blood, nutrition, night, and moonlight. The flip side or opposite of yin is yang—warm, fire, energy, activity, daytime, and sunlight. When there is yin energy deficiency that cannot be balanced with yang energy, the body will manifest relatively high (though not excessive) yang energy, and the body tends to feel warm and/or hot.

Characteristics of the Yin Deficiency Type

A typical yin deficiency type is the manifestation of a tuberculosis-like syndrome, or a menopausal-like syndrome—the tendency to feel warm, with night sweats, red cheeks, and a generally slim body structure. This type of body constitution tends to suffer constipation, dry stools, yellow urination of short duration, prone to insomnia (with special difficulty falling asleep), heart palpitations, dizziness, tinnitus, and a dry mouth even after drinking plenty of water. If the condition worsens, this person will have a dry cough without mucus, or a small amount of mucus with a trickle of blood; a cracking voice; and a feeling of pressure in the chest. Women with this type of constitution tend to have an earlier menstrual cycle than usual, with a smaller amount of dark blood. Men tend to suffer from weakness of the back and knees and pre-ejaculation, even through they may have typical or higher than normal sexual desire.

Physically, this type tends to have superficial energy in the beginning that doesn't last, and may walk and talk quickly, with an impatient manner. The body tends to feel warm, or is very sensitive to warmth, and has a lot of superficial energy and emotion, overreacting and tending to anxiety and panic attacks. Some of these types have scattered energy that makes them unable to focus on one task, after having started too many at once.

This type of body constitution tends to appear slimmer, even though they may eat more than others. They have the good fortune of being able to eat more without worrying about weight gain! It seems that their bodies can burn calories/food faster, and at the same time, they expend more energy. The activities of the body, emotional changes, and the response to the environment are all more immediate for the yin deficiency type.

Let's imagine that there is too much heat and fire in the body; the body will gradually become dry and lacking in fluids as a result of the heat activity. This is why people with this type of body constitution tend to have dry skin and wrinkles, dry mouth, dry eyes, constipation, and thin, unhealthy hair. If these signs develop and are not taken into account by modifying lifestyle in order to balance out the body, then there is the likelihood of developing hypertension, tinnitus, heart problems, insomnia, and emotional problems, such as attention deficit hyperactive disorder, anxiety, panic attacks, aggression, and mood swings from excessive heat disturbance.

How the Yin Deficiency Type Develops

For the most part, a person is born with this type of body constitution, and it cannot be changed. However, what can be done is not to exacerbate it by adding more heat and dryness to the body, and by modifying lifestyle and diet in order to keep it balanced.

Tiao Yang Methods for the Yin Deficiency Type

Choose an appropriate living environment: The yin deficient person tends to feel warm, with a dry throat and skin. This type of constitution likes to stay in the cooler weather of fall and winter, and is averse to the hot summer. Traveling high up in the mountains or going to the ocean during the summer are the best choices for this body type. As for the position of the house for this body type, it is best to reside in the north side of the house, with the door facing to the south.

The fall and winter are the seasons to nourish yin. Especially with dryness, it is important to nourish yin in the fall. First of all, stop smoking and ingesting alcohol, caffeine, hot and spicy foods, and deep-fried foods in order to preserve the body's yin and fluids. Merely drinking a lot of water is not the answer. There are many drugs and chemical additives in processed foods and supplements that can exaggerate the heat in the body, consuming more yin.

Meditation/Exercise: The best mental and emotional state for the yin deficiency type is a sense of inner peace. TCM teaches that a calm heart will preserve yin; therefore meditation is the best choice for this type of body constitution. Meditation and a calm spirit will calm down the heart fire, which preserves more yin material in the body.

Individuals with this type of body constitution should keep a well-organized work environment, keeping everything in order the best they can so that stress is reduced. Otherwise, feelings of panic and being overwhelmed will generate more fire and heat in the body. Clinically, we see people of this type who cannot fall asleep at night due to anxiety and the inability to shut their minds down after a day of too much activity and stress at work.

The best exercise for this type of body constitution is Tai Chi and Qigong, rather than competitive sports. These types should pursue hobbies that they enjoy and find soothing, such as gardening, painting, singing, and dancing.

Traditional Chinese Medicine Remedy: Acupuncture is not the best choice for this type of constitution, but rather taking an herbal formula. The traditional, patented herbal formula is Rehmannia Six. If there is more dryness in the eyes and skin, Ji Jiu Rehmannia Six (Rehmannia Six with goji berries and chrysanthemum flowers added) can be used. If there is more heat in the body, impatience, heart palpitations, tinnitus, or brief, yellow urination, one can use Zhi Po Rehmannia Six.

There are a variety of herbs that nourish yin, clear heat, and nourish the liver and kidneys' yin and blood. These include: *nu shen zi* (privet fruit, *Ligustrum*), *shan shu yu* (Asiatic Cornelian cherry), *wu wei zi* (*Schisandra* fruit), *han lian cao* (*Eclipta*), *huang jing* (*Polygonatum* rhizome), *yu zhu* (*Polygonatum*), *xuan shen* (*Scrophularia* root), goji berry, mulberry, and *mai men dong* (*Ophiopogonis* tuber).

TCM Food Therapy for Yin Deficiency

Avoid the following:
a) Hot, spicy food; alcohol; and caffeine;
b) Stimulants, drugs, and supplements for enhancing physical performance;
c) Deep-fried foods, which add more yang and heat energy.

Boiled or steamed foods, as well as fresh fruit and vegetables, are a good choice for this type of body constitution. The following food therapies should also be added into the diet for a yin deficiency type of body constitution: lily bulbs, sesame seeds, lotus seeds, fresh lotus roots (preferably juice from the young, tender lotus roots), white and black fungus mushrooms, Napa cabbage, bamboo shoots, tofu, seafood, crab meat, *Cordyceps*, and duck and pork meat (which is not warm-property meat). Fresh green tea, chrysanthemum tea, caramel tea, and mint tea are also good for this type.

Soups and Congees

Sesame congee, lily congee, bird's nest soup, pork with Napa cabbage soup, pig's feet with lilies and lotus seeds soup, black fungus mushrooms with pig's feet soup, duck with *Cordyceps*, white fungus mushrooms with lilies soup, and duck soup with ginseng and bamboo.

Or just add the following herbs to soups: *sha shen* (*Glehnia* radix), *tian men dong* (asparagus tuber), *mai men dong* (*Ophiopogonis* tuber), *shi hu* (*Ephemerantha*), *yu zhu* (*Polygonatum*), *shen di huang* (*Rehmannia* root, fresh), *di gu pi* (*Lycium* root bark), *nu zhen zi* (privet fruit, *Ligustrum*), *han lian cao* (*Eclipta*), *bie jia* (turtle shell - dorsal, Chinese Calcined) and *gui ban* (turtle shell, freshwater ventral part).

4) Qi Xu Type: Energy Deficiency

"Qi" means life force or energy, in the very narrow sense, as expressed in English. This life force is part of all life on earth, not only humans and animals, but all plants, and even the universe, which is a large Qi, giving all of life of every kind its vivid, alive appearance, its normal function, and its Shen, or spirit.

<u>How is Qi produced in the body?</u>
First of all, we have to understand that nature has a way to collect Qi (energy) from the unformed energy of both the earth and the sun, transforming it into material energy (energy as form) that we can consume, which is food. The body is then able to transform the "formed energy" (food) into an "unformed energy" (Qi), which maintains the physical body, as well as the spirit.

When we plant a seed in the earth, the seed collects the earth's Qi (energy, or the soil's nutrients), which, as unformed (nonmaterial) energy in the seed, powers the seed to transform into a sprout. After sprouting, the plant has to collect more unformed, nonmaterial energy from the universe—the air and the sunlight—for photosynthesis. It also continues to collect earth Qi, in order to totally transform the Qi into a solid form that we can touch and see, which is the food. The whole process of transformation of energy from unformed energy to formed energy for human consumption may take months, or even a year. It takes a lot of energy from both heaven and earth to nourish humans. This is why it is taught in Chinese medicine that humans are between heaven and earth, and nourished by both. If we do not protect our environment and disregard the natural laws of earth and heaven, sooner or later, human beings will be punished—something we can already see happening in certain ways.

After we consume the food (formed energy), our body has to undergo a reverse process of transforming the formed energy (food) to unformed energy that enables us to live, be active, and perform both as physical and spiritual beings. This very important organ, called the spleen, is identified as the earth element of the body in Chinese medicine. This is a totally different concept from that of the anatomic spleen in bio-medicine.

If the spleen organ is weak from birth or long-term lifestyle and diet, its function will not be preserved. As a result, food will not be transformed efficiently into energy, and the body will suffer spleen deficiency, the consequence of Qi deficiency.

Characteristics of the Qi Deficiency Type

A person with Qi deficiency feels tired and fatigues easily. Especially after a normal lunch, this type of person cannot keep his/her eyes open; after 2:00 or 3:00 p.m., there is no more energy for the body to continue to perform. These people look pale, with a sallow complexion; they speak in a low voice, with shortness of breath, and break into a spontaneous sweat very easily, with little exertion. This kind of body constitution catches colds very easily, or develops some kind of allergy. After catching a cold, this type takes a longer time to recover. Sometimes they will not even have the strength to cough, or the energy to respond verbally. Some of these people lack motivation, and may be depressed.

If there is more spleen deficiency, there may be two types of manifestations:

a) Low appetite; sallow, yellowish facial complexion; bloating and not digesting food well; watery diarrhea; muscle atrophy; and an undernourished body appearance.
b) Easily fatigued; always hungry and craving food, especially carbohydrates and junk food; a tendency to gain weight and to have loose stools or diarrhea.

If there is more kidney Qi deficiency, the person tends to retain water in the lower legs, experience pain in the heels of the feet, feel weak in the lower lumbar area, and have a tendency to urinate more frequently, with clear urine and a weak flow. In addition, some will have lower sexual desire and an inability to perform.

Causes of Qi Deficiency

Normal aging: Dr. Li Dong Yuan, a well-known doctor of Chinese medicine who lived about 800 years ago, stated that after age 35, everyone should tonify the spleen. This means that our natural human spleen starts to show deficiency around the age of 35. There are certain foods, or certain amounts of food, that the spleen can transform into energy at a younger age, but not at an older age. Modern bio-medicine has proven this statement to be right, but in a different way, and without understanding why. Bio-medicine has found that people after age 35 have a high percentage of lactose intolerance. Though it is not understood or explained in bio-medicine, Chinese medicine explains it perfectly. Dr. Li Dong Yuan founded the Spleen School and advised all doctors that they should treat and strengthen the spleen when treating any disease.

High-pressure physical activity: Professional athletes, hard physical laborers, long-term night shift workers, and long-term drug abusers repeatedly force the body to perform, putting a high demand on the body and the organs without allowing the necessary time for rejuvenation and rest. Most of these individuals have physical complaints and health problems later on, even though they may appear to still have an attractive, muscular appearance. Professional athletes in particular not only have Qi deficiency, but kidney yang deficiency; and there are no statistics to show that professional athletes have long or healthy lives because of their exhausting the vital body energy.

Constant worry and obsessive mental work: If a person is constantly worried about every little thing and does intense mental work, it will consume the body's Qi, especially at the expense of the spleen's Qi. That is why TCM teaches that the emotion of worry is the emotion of the spleen. If a person was born with this Qi deficiency constitution, he/she tends to be worried all the time, and this will continually exhaust the body's energy. Similarly, a person who is under stress, doing intense mental work, such as a student who must study hard for a big final examination, will exhaust the body's Qi (energy). As a result, the student constantly feels hungry and goes to the refrigerator to snack, putting on weight during the time of exams. This is why, in the TCM test book, it states that one with Qi Xu (energy deficiency) craves more food. With abundant Qi, one does not suffer from food cravings. For the same reason, one of the principle strategies that TCM uses to treat obesity is to strengthen spleen and Qi for long-term health and non-rebound weight control.

Tiao Yang Methods for the Qi Deficiency Type

a) Avoid Cold, Raw, or Greasy Food: In Western culture, eating cold, raw, or greasy food is very popular and widely accepted. No one stops to think that cold, raw, or greasy food may have something to do with our society of "epidemic obesity." While growing up in Chinese culture, we were constantly warned against eating cold, raw, or greasy food. It is not good for your health when you get old. When I first came to the United States, just seeing people eat in restaurants gave me culture shock: the cold drinks with ice, the platters of salad, and the big servings of fried chicken.

What's wrong with cold, raw, or greasy food?

First of all, the principles of TCM food therapy are customized according to each individual's body constitution, corresponding to seasons, age, and individual changes in body condition. There is no one diet that fits all. Cold, raw, or greasy food is neither good for everyone nor necessarily bad for everyone. But most definitely, cold, raw, or greasy food is not suitable for the Qi Xu body constitution.

Cold Food

The cold temperature of food, and food with cold properties (mostly raw vegetables, bitter melon, cucumber, mint), slows down the body's free flow of energy, especially in a digestive system that is already weak. We all know that warmth makes things open, rise, and move faster, while cold makes thing close, stagnate, and move slowly. An already weakened digestive system not only has to spend extra body energy to warm the cold food to the body's temperature, but compromises the free flow of energy in our digestive system that is needed for the transformation of food. We can see some people with weak digestive systems who tend to have diarrhea and/or stomach pain after eating cold food.

Raw Food

Raw foods, especially raw vegetables, have a cellular membrane and plant fiber that the body does not digest well, and fiber stimulates bowel peristalsis. This is why more fiber and vegetables can improve bowel movement in a normal person.

Also, the spleen (digestive system) expends more energy breaking down the cellular membrane of raw plants in order to get all the nutrients out of them. For some reason, humans do not have enough of the enzymes—unlike pandas, rabbits, horses, and cattle—that can efficiently break down, and extract nutrients from, raw plants. It is true that the raw plant is full of nutrients, some of which may be lost or damaged when cooked. However, in the Qi Xu body constitution, the spleen, or the digestive system, is weak and cannot break down or process raw plant food as a normal person might. Thus, eating raw foods tends to cause digestive system disorders. Even slightly cooking plant food by steaming it just enough to help break down the plant's cellular membrane without damaging the nutrients will provide this body type with more nutrients than eating the food completely raw.

The body's constitution can be changed by a period of lifestyle changes or after chronic disease. We understand that the body needs extra work to process raw plant food. We do not have any problem eating raw food if we have a good digestive system and eat only moderate amounts of raw food.

However, if cold, raw, and greasy food is combined together and consumed frequently, it will gradually exhaust spleen Qi over the years. Once the spleen is deficient, the body tends to gain weight.

Greasy food is phlegm itself, and phlegm will clot. If one eats greasy food with warm food and warm drink, it may not be as bad as when greasy food is taken together with cold drinks. That will consume more spleen energy and lead to more phlegm stored in the body, leading to weight gain.

Most of this type of body constitution depends on a person's lifestyle. There are some factors that depend on family history, such as obesity, hypertension, diabetes, and hyperlipidemia.

The most prominent feature of this body constitution is fatigue, with the body losing energy and tiring easily, especially after lunch and in the early afternoon. There is also the tendency to gain weight, since when the body feels fatigued, there can be a craving for carbohydrates or sweets to supplement or boost the body's energy. There may also be a sense of little motivation or drive, and the mind may lack clarity or seem unfocused.

Why does the body feel fatigued and gain weight at the same time? Why can't the body draw upon its stored energy (body fat)? The answer lies with the body's Qi, especially spleen Qi deficiency. The body needs to expend Qi (energy) from the spleen organ to process and transform food into energy for the body. When there is good stomach and spleen Qi, all the food that is consumed can be transformed for body energy use, so that we feel more energetic, have stronger immunity, with beautiful skin and hair, and we feel in good spirits. However, if we consume more food than our body can process, or our spleen Qi is weak and cannot efficiently process food consumption, even in small amounts, then the body expends its available energy processing in transforming food, rather than producing the final product: energy that the body can use. Rather, it produces the "halfway product," the phlegm (or fat, as it is called in bio-medicine).

This explains why we may feel fatigued after a big lunch; the body consumes all its energy transforming food, without any extra energy to keep you alert and functioning well. This also explains why many obese people feel fatigued all the time, as well as feeling hungry often and eating uncontrollably. It is not that the body does not have enough food, but that it is unable to produce energy from food, being forced to work to process food and only producing the incomplete product, the phlegm. As the phlegm (fat) is stored in the body under the skin, there is weight gain, fatty deposits in the blood vessels, high blood lipid levels, high cholesterol, and fatty deposits in the liver—resulting in the condition known as fatty liver.

This is why TCM treats an overweight person by strengthening the body's Qi and spleen, to enable the body to function normally and lose weight naturally, rather than enforcing diet restrictions. Forced dieting, without addressing the body's Qi and spleen condition, only leads to rebounding later, since the body's weakened energy will not have been treated, and the craving for food to provide a quick energy fix will continue.

b) Get Enough Sleep: Getting enough sleep gives the body time to rejuvenate. During yin time (nighttime), the body is set to rest, in order to restore and produce more Qi and blood for the body to perform during yang time (daytime). Sleep deprivation over a long period of time, or staying up late at night, deprives the body, depleting its Qi, blood, and yin. Sleep requirements differ according to body constitution types, age, season, and health conditions. The best time to sleep is before 11:00 p.m., which is the time of the gallbladder, according to the Chinese circadian clock of organs and meridians. Gallbladder Qi needs to be free-flowing to ensure the free flow of energy. Staying up past this time tends to make the body's Qi stagnate, making it difficult for the body to efficiently produce Qi and blood. With a good night's sleep, there will be more Qi for normal body functioning. However, a lack of sleep and Qi deficiency will cause a consistent feeling of hunger and craving for food. That is the answer to why someone under stress, who is losing sleep, tends to eat more and gain weight.

c) Moderate Exercise: The purpose of moderate exercise is to help the body move Qi and blood, in order to wake up the body's Qi so that it will transform more energy and transport the body's retained phlegm out of the body. It is important not to over-exercise, as this will exhaust the body's energy reservoirs and defeat the purpose by having the opposite result.

d) Qigong and Self-Healing: There are many kinds of Qigong exercise; seek a professional class for cultivating original Qi (kidney energy) for this body constitution. Once one learns the principle of how to cultivate the original Qi, either from a professional class or from some other source, one can make some modifications and integrate it with one's daily routine in order to balance and restore the body.

e) Other Activities: For those with this body constitution, who are easily worried or anxious, it is best to find a hobby or some activity that is enjoyable and that reduces tension with laughter, etc. If the sense of fatigue cannot be restored by resting, and worry and depression only increase, it is advisable to consult a Chinese medical doctor for acupuncture with moxibustion treatment, which can be very effective.

f) Acupuncture with Moxibustion: This is the best therapy for this type of body constitution. Herbal therapy can include *Si Jun Zi Tang*, *Shen Ling Bai Shu Wan*, or *Jing Gui Shen Qi Wan*, depending on which organ's Qi deficiency is predominant.

TCM Food Therapy for Qi Deficiency

Nourishing Qi food includes spring rice, sweet rice, millet, barley, sweet potatoes, yams, potatoes, carrots, dates, chicken, goose, rabbit, organic beef, and carp.

Examples of food therapy:

Ginseng Congee (porridge)
Ginseng: 3g, cut into very thin pieces or ground into a powder (*Dang shen* 25g can be substituted for ginseng)
Spring rice: 100g
Crystal rock sugar: a small amount

Add rice, ginseng, and water. Cook in a ceramic pot. Add rock sugar when the rice soup is cooked.

Astragalus Carp
One carp fish tail (preferably yellow-colored carp)
Astragalus: 30g
Shitake mushrooms: 20g, cut into pieces
Bamboo, cut into pieces
Fresh ginger, green onion, cooking wine, and sea salt

Brown the fish tail in a frying pan with oil first, then add all the ingredients, with water. Bring to a boil and cook 15-20 minutes until done. Take out the *Astragalus* before serving.

Eight Treasures Duck
One whole duck
Lotus seeds 50g
Yi yi ren (Job's tears) 50g,
Qian shi (Euiyale seeds) 50g

Bian dou (hyacinth bean) 50g, soaked with the other herbs in water until softened
Ham 30g, cut into small pieces
Shiitake mushrooms, cut into small pieces
Ginger and green onions, all cut into small pieces
Cooking wine, sea salt

Put all the ingredients, except for the duck, into a bowl and mix well. Put the bowl's contents into the duck stomach and sew it shut. Steam the whole duck until it is well done and almost falling apart. Serve.

5) Xue Xu Type: Blood Deficiency

Blood is a very important substance that forms life and maintains the basic physiology of life's function—the same concept as in bio-medicine. But the concept of blood in TCM goes further than this. TCM teaches that in the body's process of making blood, there are many organs involved that are working together. First of all, the spleen processes food and transforms most of the essence from food, then delivers the essence up to the heart and the lungs. The heart and lungs then transform it into red blood and pour it into the vascular system. At this point, the blood substance is finally formed and in the circulatory system. The original energy, which ensures blood formation, resides in the kidney organ. A blood deficiency body constitution can come from a chronic loss of blood, or, in most cases, from the body not producing enough blood due to a bad diet.

<u>Characteristics of the Blood Deficiency Type</u>
First of all, it must be understood that a blood deficiency body type will not necessarily produce a blood test of anemia, as would be indicated in bio-medicine. However, if a person has anemia, as pro-

duced from a blood test, one might already have signs of blood deficiency, according to a TCM diagnosis.

This type of body constitution has a sallow yellow or pale complexion and lips, heart palpations, insomnia, dizziness, low physical endurance, and sometimes, blurred vision. One may have the feeling of numbness of the limbs; a pale tongue; dry, scaly, itchy skin; dry hair that falls out easily; and pale, dry nails if the condition of blood deficiency has continued and worsened over time. Women will have scanty menstruation and be fragile, with easily provoked tendon and muscle pain and a mild tremor. Additionally, the pulse may be thin as a thread.

Tiao Yang Methods for the Blood Deficiency Type
a) **Relaxing Intense Visual Focus**: TCM teaches that intensely focusing visually on something for a long time will consume blood energy. In our modern society, with many people working on computers daily for long hours, it is common to find many who suffer from "computer syndrome," with neck, shoulder, wrist, and low back pain. Signs of blood deficiency include headaches, dizziness, blurred vision, insomnia, and a sensation of chest "fullness" from shallow breathing. What should we do when working for long periods of time on the computer? Every two hours, we should take a couple of minutes to stretch and to acupressure massage around the eyes and both sides of the head and the neck. We should also take a couple of minutes to do one or two Chinese farmer squats to stretch the low back.

Chinese Farmer Squat Exercise: Put two bare feet parallel about 2-3 inches apart. Gradually squat down, making sure that the entire soles of the feet touch the ground without lifting up, and hold for couple of minutes. This can gently stretch the lower back. Do this exercise as much as you can through the day if you have low back problems. I discovered that although

Chinese farmers work in the fields planting rice for hours and hours each day, they barely complain of back pain. I observed that when they take a break, they are always squatting down while having a conversation or eating their meals in the field. That is why the hard-working farmers rarely have low back pain, because of frequent squatting.

b) **Meditation**: People with blood deficiency often suffer mental tiredness, insomnia, and forgetfulness, and find it hard to focus. Listen to soothing, relaxing music, or watch a comedy or something lighthearted, or engage in activities that uplift the spirit, according to individual preference and interests.

c) **Avoid**: Strong coffee, strong tea, and strong alcohol, which generate heat and further consume the blood energy.

d) **Foods that Nourish Blood**: Liver (chicken, pork, goat, beef, and rabbit), beef tendon, pig heart, eggs, milk, fish, fish skin, sea cucumber, octopus, squid, black fungus mushrooms, kelp, celery, spinach, carrots, black sesame seeds, black mulberries, Chinese red dates, longan fruit, and pine nuts.

e) **TCM Herbal Formulas**: Commonly used herbal formulas for the blood deficiency body constitution include: *Dang Gui Bu Xue Tang*, *Si Wu Tang*, and *Gui Pi Tang*. If there is more fatigue, one can take *Ba Shen Tang*, *Shi Quan Da Pu Tang*, or *Ren Shen Yang Rou Tang*.

TCM Food Therapy for Blood Deficiency

There are several herbs that nourish blood energy and are usually integrated into food therapy diets. These include *shu di huang* (Rehmannia root, cooked), *dan gui* (Angelica root), *bai shao* (peony root, white), *he shou wu* (Polygonum root), *e jiao* and *ji xue teng* (Spatholobus root and vine).

Some examples of food therapy for blood deficiency:

Carrot Congee

Fresh carrots: 100g, ground or cut into very small pieces
Spring rice: 100g
Salt and mild spices to taste

Boil the carrots in water for 5 minutes. Add rice, adding in water as needed. After bringing to a boil, cook at moderate heat until done. Serve as breakfast or as soup side dish for dinner.

Function: Carrot congee is best for nourishing the blood, and for constipation due to anemia and dryness.

Longan Congee

Dried longan fruit: 15g
Spring rice: 100g
Small amount of dark brown sugar

Add water to ingredients and bring to a boil, then cook at a low temperature until the soup is done. Eat twice per week.

Function: Longan congee is best for calming the spirit, nerves, anxiety, insomnia, and forgetfulness due to blood deficiency.

Dang Gui Chicken

Dang gui (Angelica root): 30g, rinsed with water and cut into thin pieces
Astragalus: 30g, rinsed with water
One female, old organic chicken
Green onion, ginger, salt, and cooking wine

After washing the whole chicken, put the other ingredients inside the stomach. Put in a pot with water and bring to a boil. Cook at low temperature until chicken is well done and falling apart. Serve.

Function: Nourishes blood and Qi; strengthens the body. Dang Gui Chicken is best for elderly people with blood and yin deficiency and for those who are beginning the recovery process after surgery and chronic disease.

Black Force Powder
Black sesame seeds, rinsed clean and baked in a frying pan until fragrant, then crushed into powder
Wild Chinese yam: 250g, lightly baked in an oven to dry, then ground into a fine powder
He shou wu (*Polygonum* root), cut into thin pieces, lightly baked and dried in oven, then ground into a powder

Mix all three powders and seal in a glass jar. (This is the black force powder.) Taking 25 g of the black force powder, put into a cup, and pour boiling water on it while stirring to make a paste. Take once a day, for 10 days, as a course of treatment.

Function: Nourishes the blood and body essence; restores healthy hair and skin after blood deficiency. Take black force powder when the body is weak and at the beginning of the recovery process from surgery and chronic disease.

6) Qi Yu Type: Qi Stagnation

Stagnation means lack of free-flow, or blocked; Qi refers to the body's energy. If energy cannot flow freely in the body, it is just like a car accident on the freeway that causes a traffic jam. One side of the freeway is congested (a sign of excess), while the other side is empty (a sign of deficiency).

In our modern, fast-paced lifestyle, we are bombarded by stressors from many sources. Some people do not manage stress well and are easily triggered to overreact in response to stress. They manifest more physical and emotional disorders than others suffering under the same stressful conditions. This type of body constitution can be seen from childhood; this is the child that complains of having stomach pain every time he or she passes by school, or every time a certain teacher is mentioned, or refuses to eat when a person he or she perceives as unpleasant is around.

Characteristics of the Qi Stagnation Type

These people are easily agitated and quick to lose their tempers, or even become enraged under stress. The facial complexion is lackluster or pale yellow, due to a lack of good circulation. There may be dark circles around the eyes; muscle pain and tightness in the neck and shoulders; and possibly headaches or migraines, with pain that is not fixed, but moving around. Most people of this type feel fullness in the chest, and sigh a lot to release it. Worse, they may feel pressure and a dull pain in the chest. Some with this body constitution want to be alone and prefer not to associate with others, or seem to keep to themselves, walled off from everything.

The body feels warm, and hot in its core, or in the face or head (signs of congestion). However, the hands and feet feel cold (sign of deficiency) because of the stagnation and blockage of free-flow. In women, the Qi Yu body constitution type tends to have more menstrual pain, cramps, irregularity, severe premenstrual syndrome (PMS), and, believe it or not, this type of woman may even be "infertile," despite undergoing all the tests available and showing nothing identifiably wrong according to bio-medical diagnoses, texts, or case studies.

Tiao Yang Methods for the Qi Stagnation Type
1. **Exercise more, go sightseeing, and vacation to reduce stress**: Exercise increases blood and Qi circulation, opens meridians, and increases lung movement with deeper breathing. Outdoors, the energy flows more with the natural yang energy from the sun. Other kinds of exercise also reduce mental stress, such as Qigong, which uses the mind to direct the movement of Qi, or gentle movement exercise with yoga, Tai Chi, and other kinds of moderate exercise that do not further stress the body.
2. **Body Therapy**: This includes body massage, acupuncture, and acupressure. Acupuncture is the best way to reduce stress, not only for moving the body energy and blood, but for rejuvenating the stressed organs and restoring mental clarity. Most people feel a sense of well-being after acupuncture treatment. After many years of practicing TCM, I have discovered how much stress can drive people to the point of mentally breaking down and being diagnosed with some kind of mental disorder. Under psychiatric treatment, some of these stressed individuals not only do not get any help from psychiatric medication, but in fact, their behavior becomes more radical or extreme. On the opposite end, some patients lose their normal physical and mental vitality and feel and act like vegetables, without the normal range of human emotion. With several acupuncture treatments, and sometimes with only one treatment, there can be significant improvement in patients with stress and stress-related mental disorders.
3. **Other activities**: Participate in group therapy; pursue a favorite hobby; volunteer in a community event; listen to relaxing or exciting music; watch happy or funny movies. There is a Chinese saying: "Knowing you already have enough will bring happiness and peace." It tells us not to expect too much or always desire more of both power and material goods. All

those big expectations and desires not only bring stress and disease to the individual, but also many problems socially, financially, morally, and to the environment at large.
4. **Diet**: Try to avoid sugar, refined food, and coffee. Eat more green and sour-tasting foods. One can drink a moderate amount of wine, which assists in moving Qi and blood. Some foods can help move energy, such as tangerines, chives, buckwheat, garlic, dill, and ham.
5. **Herbal Therapy**: There are also some herbs that can move Qi if one has severe health problems. In this case, a TCM doctor should be consulted for evaluation.

7) Xue Yu Type: Blood Stagnation

Characteristics of the Blood Stagnation Type

This type of body constitution will result in many health problems if ignored; over the long term, it can lead to the formation of tumors and lumps in the body. The facial complexion looks dusty, without luster, almost purplish in color, with dry and fragile hair, or even hair that is falling out. The skin may be scaly and dry, and may have brown spots, with dark circles under the eyes. There may be complaints of pain in certain areas of the body; with this type, the pain is fixed, not moving around. The discomfort can be a stabbing pain or a very sharp, agonizing pain. Women may have very painful menstrual cycles with a lot of dark clots. If these women go for a long period of time without care, they may end up with uterine fibrosis, endometriosis, and/or some kind of tumor in the pelvis.

Tiao Yang Methods the Blood Stagnation Type
1. **Avoid Cold and Reduce Stress**: Cold refers to cold drinks or food, as well as not dressing warmly enough for the weather, or a living environment that is too cold for this type of individual. It is easy to imagine that if a river does not have

enough water, the river will not flow well. If there is enough water, but the riverbed has some kind of blockage, there will not be an easy flow, either. The body's blood circulation works the same way. If the body does not have enough blood or fluid (blood and yin deficiency), it will gradually stop flowing and cause blood stagnation.

Many young ladies wear very low-cut pants that show the belly button. If they dress this way during their menstrual cycle, while it may not bring immediate discomfort, later in life, they will be prone to having menstrual pain, uterine fibrosis, and even infertility, because of long-term blood stagnation caused by exposure to cold during menses. That is why TCM doctors, as well as old folks, will always advise young girls to avoid eating and drinking cold food and drink, as well as sitting on cold benches or showering in cold water during one's menstrual cycle.

On the other hand, we can imagine that if a river is blocked just as the Qi is blocked or stagnated, such as the body under long-term emotional stress, unhappiness, or physical stress, the free-flow of energy will be blocked, and the blood circulation will be comprised. That is why there is a saying in Chinese medicine, "Blood goes where Qi flows."

2. **Moderate exercises to move blood and increase circulation**: Cardiac exercise, dancing, boxing, Tai Chi, Kung Fu, Karate, and whole body massage will all increase the body's blood circulation.

3. **Meditation and Entertainment to Reduce Stress**: Blood stagnation can be caused by stress that compromises the free-flow of energy. In this case, meditation can be the best choice to integrate other stress-reduction remedies. Otherwise, stress can exaggerate blood circulation.

4. **Diet**: Moderate intake of wine can help with blood circulation. There are many foods that have the property to move blood,

such as walnuts, vinegar, bok choy, hawthorn fruit, peanuts, and black beans.
5. **Herbal Therapy:** There are many herbs with blood-moving properties that can be used in cooking, such as safflower, *di hang* (*Rehmannia* root), *dan shen* (*Salvia* root), *dang gui* (*Angelica* root), *chuang xong* (*Ligusticum wallichii radix*), *di yu* (*Sanguisorba* root), and *xu duan* (teasel root).

8) Tan Shi Type: Dampness and Phlegm

A high percentage of those with this type of body constitution are born with a family history that includes obesity, diabetes, hypertension, and hyperlipidemia. However, this type of constitution can be changed by modifying one's lifestyle through a lifelong commitment.

Characteristics of the Tan Shi (Dampness and Phlegm) Type

A person of this constitution tends to have a relatively large body structure and a square chest. The skin is damp and dusty. The body feels and acts heavy, often with dizziness; sweats easily; and has a low level of motivation. An individual with this type tends to feel fatigued and sleepy during the daytime, and a high percentage suffer sleep apnea. There is a tendency to be overweight, to bloat, and to have bowel movement problems, such as colitis, loose stools, or diarrhea, especially under stress, both physical and emotional.

With a fatigued body, by the end of the day there will be mild swelling of the lower legs around the ankles, with pitted edema. Many of this type suffer a certain degree of depression; many develop allergies, with sinus allergy a common ailment, as well as allergies to foods, with the possibility of having skin problems. All signs and symptoms will be exaggerated during damp weather and in a damp location, such as a damp work environment, and by the consumption of food that generates dampness, such as dairy products, fatty foods, fine carbohydrates, and sugar.

Some have body odor and more discharge from the body, such mucus, leucorrhea, and sweat, along with a dusty or lackluster skin complexion. No matter how often the face is cleaned or a commercial facial performed, the complexion will never shine so long as there is dampness accumulating in the body.

If dampness and phlegm stay in the body for long, another sub-type of body constitution will develop: dampness-with-heat constitution. The body will then have more of a yellow-colored discharge, whether from sweating, nasal discharge, or vaginal discharge, and will have a strong odor when urinating and defecating. This type of constitution will have a significant impact on the health and appearance of the skin. The facial complexion looks dirty, greasy, and lackluster, with larger pores. If there is acne, it tends to become badly infected, with painful red boils filled with pus, as well as blackheads. Some of the dampness-with-heat body constitution types have chronic skin lesions on the lower legs and ankles, and, as I've seen clinically, pitted edema, dark discoloration, and thickened skin with dry, yellow, odorous, uneven crusts that last for many years. Should I look at the tongue of this type, it will look moist and puffy, covered with a greasy, yellow coating.

We all know that dampness and phlegm are heavy and sticky by nature, so this means that this condition is relatively more difficult to treat. More importantly, it must be recognized and identified, followed by a change of lifestyle to prevent it from getting worse.

Tan Shi Body Constitution and an Unhealthy Lifestyle

Everyone understands that our body is mostly composed of water. The water in our bodies carries fresh nutrients to all parts of the body, and at the same time, dissolves all the waste to be discharged via sweating, urination, breathing, spit, and of course, defecation. Just as there is a way to take in water and fluids, there must be a way for it to be discharged in order to keep balance in the body. To maintain a balance, all the organs must work together, consuming the body's energy in the process. When the body starts to accumulate phlegm, or even show signs of accumulating dampness, there will be mucus in the throat, sinuses, or respiratory system; swollen joints, or accumulation of water under the skin; cloudiness in the urine; and mucus in the stool. All the visible mucus, dampness, and phlegm are called "substantial phlegm" in TCM. However, there is a slight difference between dampness and phlegm. Phlegm comes from a long period of unsolved dampness, so that it becomes more condensed. This means that once the body has phlegm, it is harder to treat than when it is at the stage of dampness.

Besides the substantial phlegm that we can see, as mentioned above, there is the more dangerous phlegm that we cannot see, the insubstantial phlegm—phlegm that can travel and become lodged in different parts of the body's organs. With insubstantial phlegm deposited under the skin, we gain weight and eventually become obese. If it deposits in the liver, we develop fatty liver. If deposited in the heart, it will cause a heart attack, stroke, and hyperlipidemia. In other words, insubstantial phlegm is what modern bio-medicine calls "fat."

There are three important organs in charge of the body's water metabolism: the spleen, the lungs, and the kidneys. Of these three, the most important is the spleen. As mentioned before, if the spleen does not function well, or if we eat too much food that taxes the limits of the spleen's processing capacity, then this food cannot be turned into energy that we can use, but becomes an incomplete product: phlegm. For this reason, if we eat greasy or sweet food for a late dinner, the next day we will definitely notice that there is phlegm and mucus in the throat.

There is a saying in TCM, "The spleen generates phlegm, and the lungs store it." Lung energy is in charge of the respiratory system, including the trachea, bronchi, throat, nasal passages, and sinuses, as well as being in charge of the skin that provides special defensive energy to protect against pathogen invasion. Once the spleen is deficient and cannot support lung energy, the phlegm will be generated and distributed from the spleen to the lungs, and there will be sinus allergies, sinus congestion, post-nasal discharge/drip, and skin lesions. Why does the spleen have an impact on the lungs? The spleen's function in the body is just like the earth element for humans. It transforms energy, starting from a seed and developing into a mature plant, crop, tree, or whole root for human consumption. According to the five elements, the earth (the spleen) will generate metal (the lungs). Once the spleen is weak, it not only cannot produce enough energy to support the lungs, but will also generate phlegm, which congests the lungs.

As we can imagine, if a river is blocked, it forms a pond. Since the water in the pond cannot flow, it cannot be refreshed, and gradually the stagnant pond water will become rancid. The same is true for the body: if the dampness and phlegm stagnate for too long, it will become rancid and form toxins, pus, and congealed lumps. The dampness-with-heat type of body constitution is at a high risk of forming a lump with toxins: cancer.

Tiao Yang Methods for the Tan Shi Type

1. Try to avoid living and working in a damp, moist, rainy environment.
2. Moderate exercise will invigorate the body and the spleen to transform phlegm.
3. People with the Tan Shi constitution should avoid food that generates phlegm and dampness, such as greasy food, dairy, refined carbohydrates, sugar, and any other processed food that contains preservatives and additives. Try to avoid too much cold and raw food, which compromises the spleen organ energy and easily results in more production of phlegm in the body.
4. Avoid excess salt intake. Some foods have properties that help drain dampness, prevent phlegm, and cause weight loss, such as turnips, water chestnuts, seaweed, jellyfish, onions, small red beans, mung beans, lava beans, pearl bar-

ley (coix seeds), white beans, and Chinese red dates.

TCM Food Therapy for the Tan Shi Type

Tangerine and Ginger Tea

    Both dried tangerine peels and ginger can assist in transforming and eliminating dampness in the spleen; they are also used to alleviate phlegm caused by spleen deficiency. Tangerine peels and ginger counterbalance each other, and are commonly used in everyday cooking in China. One can use dried tangerine peels in tea as well, giving an aromatic taste to dry mucus and dampness.

Coix Seeds (Pearl Barley) Tea

    Coix seeds are a common grain used in Chinese cuisine. They are also used as an herb to dry dampness, to drain water from the lower part of body, and to make the knees more flexible in older age. They can also be made into a tea by soaking them in water overnight and then slowly cooking until soft. Then simply drink the liquid as a tea. Most Chinese people use coix seeds along with other kinds of legumes and rice to make congee for breakfast or soup to be eaten with the dinner meal.

Mung Bean Soup

    Mung beans are not only an excellent food to drain dampness; they also clear heat and toxins in the body. They are best for clearing damp heat and summer heat. Simply soak the mung beans in water until they become soft, and then cook until they open, adding a little crystal rock white sugar. This is a great natural drink for detoxifying the body, clearing a mild summer heat stroke, and most importantly, clearing pesticides from the body after eating contaminated food.

Bai Bian Dou **(Hyacinth Bean, "Flat Bean")**

    This is a type of white-colored bean used primarily in herbal formulas for drying dampness and dampness-related diarrhea. Use 30-50g of hyacinth bean and rice to make rice soup.

Kelp and Seaweed

Both of these not only drain dampness in the body, but also act like blood filters. Kelp and seaweed can also expel/flush out all toxins from the digestive system.

Hawthorn Fruit

This special, sour-tasting fruit grows mostly in mountainous areas in northern China. It is consumed as a fruit when fresh, and a tea when dried. It is a great aid in digesting fatty foods and meat, in lowering cholesterol and triglycerides, and in preventing heart disease.

Lotus Leaf Tea

Lotus leaves are widely used as an herb to drain dampness, clear summer heat, and help in weight loss. They can be used in their dried form to make tea. In the countryside of China, the fresh, whole leaves are used in the summer for cooking. When making rice soup, whole, fresh lotus leaves are used as a lid to cover the boiling soup, touching the broth as it cooks. The rice turns a light green color and absorbs the natural fragrance of the lotus leaves. Eat it for breakfast and as a soup with dinner.

Certain Vegetables

Some vegetables that are very good to dry dampness are winter melon, cucumbers, celery, and Napa cabbage.

Others

Green tea, honeysuckle tea, and dried loquat leaf tea are also good for this type.

TCM Herbal Therapy for the Tan Shi Type

If the Dampness/Phlegm body constitution type has signs of allergies, skin lesions, and swelling, and/or begins to feel a sense of heaviness and gains weight, an herbal formula, such as *Shen Ling Bai Shu San*, should be taken to strengthen the spleen and drain dampness, or a TCM doctor should be seen for consultation and treatment.

Chapter 8
Food Therapy for Natural Detoxification

What are toxins?

We all have heard talk of toxins and detoxification. Toxins in the body are not the poisons that we usually talk about, which can kill us immediately. Much commercial advertising and different business groups stress that we are living in a very toxic environment with contaminated food, polluted water and air, and many artificial, synthetic products of all kinds in our lives, from household detergents to food additives, and even in our daily vitamin supplements. Of course, all this bad news of toxic exposure permeating our lives is real. But these profit-driven companies don't tell the other side of the story—that the body has the natural ability to detoxify itself.

Instead, these companies and marketers use only some of the facts to create a sense of psychological threat, using it as a pitch like politicians in order to sell their products and create the illusion that they are here "to save the day." Because of this, there are hundreds of detoxification gurus, programs, and elixirs sprouting up like mushrooms, with harsh methods and "therapies" that ignore the uniqueness of each person's condition. The goal is to make people buy into the notion that the body can detoxify only through these programs they are peddling. Of course, we are living in a money-driven society that profits from putting people in a panic, making them ready to pay for any detoxifying method. People spend thousands of dollars for high-dose supplements that actually overload and deplete the organs' energies, rather than supporting or detoxifying them. There are many cases of people who undergo harsh, so-called detoxifying or cleansing procedures that end up exhausting the body for weeks or months before they are able to recover their prior state.

We have to understand our bodies and many related factors in order to choose a proper detoxification method.

1) Detoxification of the body should be a long-term process and a lifestyle choice. Some people depend on intermittent detoxification programs and taking commercial detoxification supplements once in a while, rather than committing to long-term lifestyle changes. However, subjecting the body to one-time programs or methods that detoxify the body through harsh cleansings is not the way to health. It takes commitment to change our daily routine and diet habits. So long as you eat and your body is still alive and your cells are still working, your body will continually produce wastes every second. The body has to discharge this waste through its own natural methods, such as breathing, urination, sweating, and defecation.

2) Detoxifying the body can be done the natural way at home. For extreme cases, one can participate in a detoxification program, but it should be followed up with healthy lifestyle changes and a balanced diet to maintain body wellness.

3) The body has the capacity to work and balance itself in the process of self-protection and detoxification. We have to understand that no matter what kind of life form on the planet we are talking about—plants, microbes, animals, or humans—as long as life continues, there has to be a way to consume nutrients to support growth, as well as a way to discharge wastes. This process must follow its own biological parameters, keeping itself in balance in order to sustain life. The body will stop functioning properly if there is a rapid interruption of biological balance, whether from the external environment or internally, or if the body's signals are ignored and inappropriate programs or modalities are used to override the body's natural negative feedback mechanism for adjusting imbalance and thereby countering its natural laws.

One of the fundamental differences between Western medicine and Traditional Chinese Medicine is that TCM tries to restore the body to its own maximum capacity to enable it to work and perform, rather than "supplementing" the body. While supplements can be beneficial in certain cases, for many health conditions, supplement therapy will take over or shut down the body's own natural functioning. This is because the supplements—hormones, drugs, and/or mechanical methods—cover up the "negative signal" to the body, and as a result, the body loses its feedback mechanism that tells it to self-regulate, or restore itself back to normal homeostasis.

For example, in long-term abusers of laxatives, or those who depend on colonic therapy for bowl movements, the body not only loses its own peristaltic rhythm as it is totally overridden or disabled by an external force, but the GI mucosal lining loses its ability to absorb nutrients. Long-term abuse of laxatives locally stimulates the bowel for a bowel movement, shutting down the body's own nervous system that sends the impulse (or signal by neutron transmitter). This signal is not only to assist the bowel's regular peristalsis, but to maintain a healthy mucosal lining of the GI system. The mucosal lining becomes thin, with many brown spots, and malfunctions after long-term laxative abuse. TCM believes that using laxatives will exhaust the spleen and stomach Qi and will lead to compromising the body's defensive Qi (immunity). Once spleen is deficient, the body will lose muscle mass, and many other health problems will follow.

4) Fasting and colon cleansing are not appropriate for everyone. These detoxification methods should only be used with moderation under certain conditions.

Where are the toxins coming from?

Internal toxins

These so-called "toxins" come from normal metabolites in the food that we consume, especially protein, fat, and additive-enriched food. These metabolites must remain under a certain level in order not to interrupt the body's normal functioning. For example, the body needs glucose at a certain level in the blood in order to maintain functioning. If glucose levels in the blood reach a high level, then the level of glucose becomes toxic to the body, which can lead to coma. The same thing applies to uric acid, a normal metabolite from protein. When it reaches a certain level, it can cause gout and form stones in the body. Then the normal waste becomes toxic. Besides these, there are many other chemical wastes generated from all corners of the body, such as nitric acid, SO_3, and carbon dioxide, all of which can be called "internal toxins" when their accumulation threatens and ages the body. So the metabolite waste and toxins are basically the same thing in the body, according to the concentrations inside the body.

The toxins in the body are "unformed toxins" that cannot be directly seen. Once the toxins accumulate to the point that a localized redness, swelling, or even a lump forms, then they become "formed toxins" that we can directly see. We will feel warm, with a heat sensation if there are unformed toxins accumulating in the body. That is why Chinese medicine calls unformed toxins "heat."

Food can be classified as having cooling, cold, warm, or hot properties in TCM. The classifications are mostly based on the interactions between the body and food. Food with neutral or slight cooling, or slightly warm properties, is easily digested and transformed. This means it does not consume too much of the body's energy in its normal assimilation, or in other words, there is not much heat (toxin) produced during the process. On the other hand, other kinds of food require the body to work hard to digest, transform, and assimilate it, which means the food is not compatible with the body. The harder the food is for the body to break down, the more energy it must consume to process it, and the more waste that will be generated and the more heat the body will produce. When heat accumulates to a certain level, signs of toxicity in the body will manifest.

In Chinese culture, people know to eat more cooling foods in order to counteract "heat" in the body. All these cooling, or cold, herbs and vegetables carry detoxification, or natural antibiotic properties. These foods include dandelion, honeysuckle, chrysanthemum flowers, mint, bitter melon, and cucumbers. If the body cannot break down what we eat, it is difficult to assimilate and transform the food into the body. In other words, instead of consuming the food for energy, the body cannot utilize the food, and excess heat is generated as it tries to process it. Most people find that food that strongly disagrees with them will cause some kind of allergic reaction or panic response, or that the body will try to eliminate it in some kind of dramatic way. This dramatic elimination process—such as spiking a high fever, breaking out in a rash, or the skin tearing away from the body—can be catastrophic to the body and disrupt normal organ function, as with asthma, diarrhea, Johnson's reaction (in which the mucus and skin of the whole body is damaged), and even going into shock or lapsing into a coma.

This is why TCM food therapy predominantly uses natural cooling herbs and plants, such as celery, bitter melon, and cucumbers, to clear the condition of excess heat in the body (or as described by biomedicine, acidic and toxic conditions). It should be mentioned that alcohol, strong coffee, and cigarette smoking all generate heat in the body, both in the short- and long-term. To reduce heat, watch what you eat, eat balanced meals with cooling and warm foods according to your body's condition, and avoid processed foods.

External toxins

External toxins can include polluted or chemically treated water, air, or soil; as well as food sources, such as sodas, other beverages, canned or preserved food, and the artificial color found in sweets. There are so many chemical products in our daily lives that we become "addicted" to them, such as with household detergents, personal soaps and body products, household and garden pesticides, cosmetics, plastic products, paints, and electrical devices that emit a magnetic field. All of these products should be used with caution. Certain plants and flowers, such as water lilies and poinsettias, should not be in the bedroom during sleep because of their toxicity. Heavy metals, such as mercury, lead, silver, and gold, inactivate cellular enzymes, which can cause cell apoptosis. All of these chemicals directly impact the body, which is unable to process them. Remember that external toxins can kill human beings in a very short time. In our society, the most common sources of toxic poisoning comes from medications, overdosing with supplements, and substance abuse.

Stress

Stress can cause great harm, both physically and emotionally. If stress overrides the body's balance, it will compromise the body's Qi and free blood flow, resulting in more production of toxins and their accumulation in the body. According to bio-medicine, when people are under stress from both internal and external sources, the sympathetic nervous system will be affected. This in turn triggers the adrenal glands to secrete stress hormones, which include:

- **Cortisone**
  This hormone deals effectively with acute conditions, but at the expense of the immune system, since, in response to stress, cortisone breaks down immune system proteins with metabolites. Additionally, cortisone increases fatty tissue deposits, with the body retaining more sugar for quick energy to help deal with the stressful condition. Therefore, people experiencing chronic, long-term stress will have lower immunity and will generally gain weight.

- **Aldosterone**
  This hormone increases water and salt retention, so that people under chronic stress are prone to hypertension and edema.

- **Androgen**
  Women under long-term stress typically have irregular menstrual cycles, grow unwanted hair, have painful PMS, and have difficulty becoming pregnant due to the excess secretion of androgen.

- **Adrenal medulla hormones**
  These hormones include epinephrine and non-epinephrine hormones, known as the "fight or flight hormones" that help us quickly respond to urgent situations. Adrenal medulla hormones cause all the peripheral arteries to contract, raising blood pressure and heart rate. Under conditions of acute stress, it is common to turn pale, have a headache and tightness in the stomach, and cold hands and feet. With chronic, long-term stress, there is the likelihood of high blood pressure, heart disease, and stroke.

The Vagus Nervous System (parasympathetic nervous system) counteracts the sympathetic nervous system to help balance out stress. When activated, visceral blood vessels dilate, and the visceral organs increase their blood flow, rejuvenating the body. The peripheral arterial and facial muscles relax; there is increased circulation to the skin; blood pressure returns to normal; and the heart rate stabilizes. Since the parasympathetic nervous system is taken over by the sympathetic nervous system when the body is stressed, in order to reduce stress, the sympathetic nerve impulses must be reduced, the vagus nerve toned, and the parasympathetic nerve impulses increased.

Stress is one of the most common factors leading to many of the health problems, both physical and emotional, in our society. Stress-related health problems have been increasing dramatically in America and already surpass indicators in Japan, once believed to have the most stressed workforce on earth. The average American works 60 hours per week, and unfortunately, there are few stress-reduction and prevention programs offered in our medical system. Stress is not a traditional bio-medicine "diagnosis" or condition, and since stress cannot be seen with x-ray, MRI, regular blood testing, or other traditional diagnostics, and diagnosis in bio-medicine is based on test evidence, there is no chapter dedicated to stress in Western medical texts.

Stress cannot be classified as solely an internal or external factor that makes the body produce toxins. Most causes of stress come from external factors, but it must be taken into consideration that the internal body system reacts to external stressors, causing physical and mental imbalance. In reality, we cannot always change external stressors, but we can make changes internally to deal with stress better. Mostly, this internal change comes from the power of the mind, and internally balancing our organs and energy, such as with meditation, exercise, Tai Chi, Qigong, and yoga. And, not yet known to many, acupuncture may be the best choice for managing stress.

How does TCM explain how stress causes the body to accumulate toxins?

Imagine that the body has a lot of Qi (energy) flowing to every part of the body and organs through many channels called meridians. Stress is like an external force that constricts these meridians, causing body energy and circulation blockages. TCM calls this "Qi stagnation." This can be understood as similar to when one is watering the garden and accidentally steps on the hose, restricting the flow of water and causing a blockage. At the point of blockage, there will be an accumulation of waste and toxins, since they cannot be properly transported and discharged from the body. Common examples are the experience of constipation when under stress; a feeling of pressure in the chest; a headache with a warm sensation; or facial acne—all indications of the accumulation of heat/toxins due to a blockage in the body. Imagine the water hose again, with pressure (stress) on one side of the blockage/congestion, but the other side remaining empty, without water. So it is with the body. On the side of the blockage, the organs and peripheral areas and skin are not nourished and not functioning normally because of a lack of circulation of Qi and blood. There will follow experiences of cold hands and feet, a duller complexion, or a digestive system unable to process food, which manifests as diarrhea or loose stools. For those suffering under long-term stress, this can lead to heart ischemia, heart attack, and stroke.

Detoxification and Longevity in TCM

In Chinese medicine, it is believed that detoxification is an important part of promoting longevity, and that detoxification can restore youthfulness, ensure skin beauty and free-flowing energy, and enlighten the spirit. In China, detoxifying the body is associated with well-being, natural beauty enhancement, and longevity.

How Toxins Cause the Body to Stop Functioning Properly

<u>Digestive Disorders and Fatigue Syndromes</u>
A healthy body is like a well-designed holistic system that transforms the energy in food to an energy form (Qi) that the body can use. The energy travels throughout the circulatory system to the organs and tissues, which perform and work synergistically. It collects and discharges wastes from every corner of the body. The body discharges solid wastes through the digestive system, with the less-solid and liquid toxins being absorbed into the bloodstream after being filtered by the liver. The kidneys and the skin also discharge waste in liquid form.

Carbon dioxide from the system is discharged from the lungs. The body is smart enough to know how much it has to work to detoxify or discharge the toxins that it makes each day in order to keep a balanced inner environment. However, the body has a limit to its capacity. If, for whatever reason, there is an excess of toxins in the body, and the body's capacity to eliminate them is overcome, then it will begin to have problems. The body will then begin to show signs of fatigue, having exhausted its energy fighting and discharging toxins. Other signs can include bad breath, bloating, constipation and ulcers—all indications of toxic accumulation in the digestive system.

Obesity

One of the reasons that we may gain weight is that the body cannot keep up with the elimination of waste, phlegm, and other toxins. The body may be too weak to transform and transport waste from the body—TCM calls this "spleen deficiency"—or the body may be overloaded with toxins and overextended in its capacity to eliminate them. If, as in the first instance, the body is too weak to perform its normal function of transforming energy from food, the resulting lack of energy production will be fatigue, as well as giving the body a false feeling of needing more food. This sets off food/energy cravings for a quick fix of carbohydrates, sweets, energy bars, energy drinks, and/or pre-packaged junk food—all food products that enjoy an abundant market, unfortunately.

This false feeling of hunger is an indicator that the body does, in fact, lack energy, but not because we do not supply it with enough food. Rather, it is because the body's organ system (the spleen system) is too weak to process food to make energy for the body. At the same time, as we supply more food to the body due to our false hunger, the already weakened body is again overloaded with food it cannot fully process to create useable energy. Therefore, more "halfway" products from the food will be produced and stored in the body as fat, or as TCM calls it, "phlegm."

This is a summary of the vicious cycle that results in the accumulation of toxins and obesity. It is also the process of the body expending its energy to detoxify itself due to an unhealthy lifestyle of trying to relieve false hunger with quick energy foods loaded with sugar, fat, and what are ultimately toxins that the body cannot fully digest. The end result is that the body accumulates more and more stagnant phlegm (fat), with a host of toxins contained in the fat, ultimately becoming obese. The more toxins the body accumulates, the more body function will decline, and the more weight the body will gain.

Body Pain

Many forms of toxins can accumulate in the body, such as uric acid found in gout disease, phlegm accumulation in the joints, or phlegm (cholesterol) accumulation inside the blood vessels. These cause blockage of energy flow and blood circulation. Chinese medicine teaches that where there is blockage, there is pain. This is why TCM treats pain with acupuncture to unblock the meridians, and herbs as an antidote to the toxins.

Aging

In balanced homeostasis, when the body has enough nutrients and is free of harmful toxins, the body rejuvenates properly and is fully functional. On the other hand, a toxic environment in the body can alter and damage cells and body tissues. TCM teaches that the most basic foundation for any life form starts with Qi and blood. If, for any reason, Qi and blood cannot be rejuvenated or circulated, then there is stagnation and accumulation of toxins, and life will be diminished. An unbalanced body, physically or emotionally, will result in accelerating the aging process.

Immune System Decline

When one of the body's defensive systems, which we call the

immune system, is compromised, there will follow many allergies, immune system disorders, susceptibility to infection, and the growth of cancer cells. A well-known maxim in TCM from thousands of years ago is that if the body's defensive system is intact, there will be no disease. Throughout TCM history, the TCM doctor's main strategy for dealing with health problems has been to focus on strengthening the body's Qi to prevent disease. In fact, as modern research indicates, a normal individual has millions of cells that become abnormal and even cancerous every day as the body maintains its normal function of regenerating and repairing tissue. At the same time, however, it has millions of immune cells, such as lymphocyte CD8, CD4, NK (natural killing) cells, and macrophages to recognize and destroy the abnormal and cancerous cells before they can develop into tumors.

Degenerative Disease

Tissue that is damaged and aged by toxins over a long period of time will decline in its function and capacity to rejuvenate itself, followed by degenerative disease.

Skin Problems

Skin is one of the body's organs; the only difference is that it is an external organ that we can directly see. If our internal organs are not balanced, or there are too many toxins in the body, our skin, like a mirror, will reflect these internal conditions. Also, the skin, by sweating, is one of the most important detoxifying organs. If there are too many toxins in the body, the skin must work harder to detoxify, and through this process it will change texture and appearance, reflecting what is happening internally. After many years of smoking, the skin will become dry and wrinkled, along with dryness of the organs and the throat, which leads to a lack of vital fluid and moisture and changes in the voice.

Alcohol can generate heat (toxins) in the body, especially in the liver and stomach systems. With long-term abuse of alcohol, there will be skin redness, often observed in the center of the face, and appearing along the stomach meridian on the face. Once the liver accumulates too many toxins from alcohol abuse or other sources, the skin will look dull or lackluster from aging, or will develop brown spots in certain areas of the body and face. Pale, sallow skin and/or a darkening of the complexion indicate deficiency or stress in the body. An experienced TCM doctor can get a lot of information related to one's health condition from observation of the complexion. This is why new patients coming to my clinic will be asked not to wear any makeup or concealers that cover the true facial complexion. For beautiful skin and to maintain skin treatments and/or facials, patients must also address their underlying health problems and contributing lifestyle choices. Some of my patients are pleasantly surprised with their skin changes after treating and balancing the inner organs, when they hadn't intended to treat the skin.

The Body's Natural Detoxification Systems

As long as the body maintains its normal metabolic function, it will continue to process, absorb, assimilate, and break down the food we eat. We all know that this metabolic process also entails generating a lot of waste as part of its normal function. Still, it is unusual for anyone to need a daily detoxification regimen in order to maintain a healthy life. This is because, through the evolutionary process, the body has developed the remarkable, sophisticated, and versatile capacity to survive in a naturally hostile environment. This includes an organ system with the natural capability to detoxify and maintain inner balance. Following the laws of nature and the natural rhythms of the body, the principle of detoxification should focus on restoring the body's own capacities and functions in order to reach the goal of balance and longevity. It is not advisable to risk seriously disrupting the body's own natural balancing systems with experimental commercial procedures, supplements, or extreme diets, all of which could easily do more harm than good.

1. The Digestive System
   a) <u>Bowel movements</u>: The most important method the body uses to detoxify itself is by discharging wastes and toxins. When we consume food, chewing it well, it is transported to the stomach, where stomach acids assist in digestion, also killing bacteria in the process. Afterward, the food is transported to the small intestine, where most of the chemical digestion takes place. Most of the digestive enzymes that act in the small intestine are secreted by the pancreas. These enter the small intestine in order to digest food, and also to kill bacterial microbes, so there is still a relatively low level of bacteria in the small intestine.

      Absorption of the majority of nutrients takes place in the jejunum (the middle section of the small intestine), although iron is absorbed in the duodenum (the first section of the small intestine). Vitamins and bile salts are absorbed in the terminal ileum (the last section of the small intestine). The small intestine in an adult is, on average, about five meters (16 feet) long, with a normal range of 10-22 feet, so that each person's absorption period in the small intestine is unique. It is not wise to use extreme, harsh methods to force bowel movements as a result of interruption of the food absorption period. It might be normal for one individual to have a bowel movement once every other day; another may have one up to twice a day—all being considered normal, so long as it is regular.

      The waste will then pass through the ileocecal valve into the large intestine, which houses over 700 species of bacteria that perform a variety of functions. These bacteria also produce large amounts of vitamins, especially vitamin K and biotin, for absorption into the blood. However, if there are too many undigested polysaccharides, especially food not being digested and absorbed well as a result of using laxatives, following fermentation by the bacteria, there will be production of toxic by-products, such as nitrogen, carbon dioxide, hydrogen, methane, and hydrogen sulfide. The interaction of these toxins can cause gas (flatulence).

If, for some reason, the large intestine's normal bacterial flora become imbalanced, such as from using antibiotics or a lowered immunity due to other causes, there will more toxins produced in the GI system, along with weak absorption and lowered production of vitamins. TCM believes that overnight stagnation of the stool in the colon produces most of the body's toxins. Maintaining regular bowel movements is one of the most important methods for the body to get rid of toxins. However, this does not necessarily mean that we should use external means to force the body to have a bowel movement, since interrupting the body's own bowel movement rhythm only results in causing more harm to the body. If one is having difficulty and has a special health condition, or is elderly, a natural and gentle method to assist one's bowel movement should be used, as can be found with many folk remedies.

b) <u>Vomiting</u>: Vomiting is a self-protection reflex, although it is not the usual method for the body to detoxify. It is only in certain conditions that vomiting is the first line of protection for the body, such as the intake of unclean food or chemicals that are imminently dangerous to the body. In extreme conditions, such as liver and/or kidney failure, when all of the body's systems are overwhelmed by an overload of toxins, vomiting can assist the body in discharging toxins.

2. The Kidneys

Urination is another important natural detoxification method used by the body. It is a sophisticated system to balance fluid, PH, minerals, and electrolytes. The body needs a minimal amount of fluid to dilute and transport waste from the body in liquid form. If one is in the habit of not drinking enough water, and high concentrations of urine stay in the bladder and urethra tube for long periods of time, not only does this harm bladder tissue and increase the chances of cancer, but it also increases the chance of forming kidney and/or bladder stones. It is important to drink more water to dilute toxins and to discharge urine to avoid harming the urinary tract and maintain healthy tissue that is free from infection. At the same time, there is a lot of confusion as to how much water one should drink as a rule. There is no single standard amount that fits every individual, with their differing professions, body types, responses to the different seasons, etc. There is a lot of controversy about how much water we should consume to maintain optimum health. It depends on many factors, such as body mass, gender, profession, how much normal daily perspiration there is, and how much water is consumed along with meals. There is an old saying in TCM: "If you want to live long, keep your urine clear all day long." The color of a healthy individual's urine is an indicator of whether the body has enough water.

3. The Respiratory System

Coughing and deep breathing both can be considered detoxification. Regular breathing is a normal physiological process of the body for detoxifying. Coughing is one of the body's defensive methods. If there is something in the respiratory system that causes blockage and irritates the airways, the body must cough it up in order to clear a pathway. However, chronic chemical exposure, or allergens stimulating the respiratory system with constant coughing, can cause lung problems. When under stress or intensely concentrating on some task, we tend to hold our breath or take shallow breaths.

Shallow breathing can have several negative impacts on the body:

a) Instead of the maximum CO_2/O_2 exchange in the lungs, there is only a partial exchange. The capacity of the lungs to inhale to full expansion and exhale to maximum deflation is not exercised. People complain every day of headaches and a warm facial sensation at the end of a stressful workday, caused by too much accumulation of CO_2 in the body. It is important to remember to do some deep breathing once a while to overcome this problem.

b) Deep breathing is a way to facilitate the circulation of Qi and blood throughout all the internal organs and beneath the body's surface. TCM believes that one aspect of the lung Qi is called "defensive" Qi. Defensive Qi needs to circulate throughout the body surface in order to protect it from pathogens. There is a saying in TCM: "The lung acts as a canopy over all the vessels of the body."

c) Deep breathing is a way to gently massage the abdominal organs and assist in energy flow to the organs and throughout the body to detoxify. When the lungs are maximally expanded at the end of inhalation, the diaphragm is pushed downward, creating pressure on the organs in the abdomen and pelvis. This helps to ease the congestion of the abdominal organs and enhances circulation in the lymphatic and vein systems. When the lungs are maximally deflated at the end of exhalation, the diaphragm will return upward, leaving more space and negative pressure on the abdomen and pelvis, allowing for new, fresh blood circulation to the organs.

This is how slow, deep breathing exercises can help reduce body stress and refresh and nourish the organs. Qigong therapy teaches you to visualize your breath going into the nose with inhalation, directly to the *Dan tian* area (around the abdominal umbilical area), opening and circulating Qi via all the organs. The exhalation travels up the energy channel—called the Ren meridian—up the front and center of the body;

from the genitals, up through the lower, middle, and upper abdomen; and continuing up the chest all the way to the center of the neck/throat and out the mouth.

4. The Liver

In bio-medicine, besides synthesizing a variety of proteins, antibodies, stored vitamins, starches, fat, and blood, the liver is also an important organ for filtering toxins and deactivating chemicals—from external sources like drugs, or from substances absorbed from an internal source of bio-waste. In TCM, however, when liver Qi is stagnant, it manifests more on an emotional level, with symptoms like impatience, irritability, and being easily angered. This condition is called liver Qi stagnation. If liver Qi does not flow freely, signs and symptoms can subsequently manifest on the physical level, with body pain, headaches, elevated blood pressure, insomnia, digestive system disorders, and PMS for women, depending on the length and severity of the liver Qi stagnation. Since Qi is the energy that assists in blood circulation, blood stasis will follow when Qi stagnation goes on for too long. The body will then experience a stable, fixed pain, menstrual difficulty, skin discoloration, and even the formation of tumors, if the stagnation of Qi and blood continues over a long period of time. Bio-medicine and TCM agree that liver detoxification should include both physical (dietary) and emotional components.

5. The Skin

The skin detoxifies the body with its function of perspiration, thus discharging body wastes and toxins from the lymphatic system underneath the skin, as well as cleansing the skin. Chinese medicine believes that sweating is a natural process conducted by Qi flow to the skin surface. When Qi flows, the blood follows. Thus, sweat is called "the fluid of the blood" and is the natural process for blood cleansing. When Qi and blood flow freely to the skin surface, there is no blockage, and the whole body is protected from pathogens.

The skin has the capacity to assist the body in regulating water, balancing electrolytes, and discharging waste from the body. The body's defensive Qi is consumed during the process of sweating, so excessive sweating will exhaust Qi. However, the body will not feel exhausted from normal sweating. The skin works harder to rid itself of excessive wastes when we suffer from certain medical conditions such as liver or kidney failure, when there is more accumulation of waste. Toxins discharged via sweat carry an odor and irritate the skin.

According to TCM, perspiration is a process to expel pathogens. When the body has a cold with fever; without sweating, the body aches; after promoting sweating, the pathogen is expelled, the body feels less pain, and the fever is gone. However, there is a limit to how much one should sweat for treatment purposes, according to the individual. An experienced TCM doctor has to know how to strengthen and supplement the body's defensive Qi that becomes exhausted during the sweating process. This is why many patients suffering from influenza, who are treated by a TCM doctor, will discover that all their symptoms will improve, or even clear up immediately. The promotion of sweating without regard to individual body constitution or current health conditions only does harm. At the menopausal stage of life, it is common to see women with signs of dry throat and skin, hot flashes, heart palpitations, insomnia, mood swings, and constipation. These all indicate kidney water energy deficiency, according to a TCM diagnosis. For this condition of the body, the promotion of sweating will cause the body to lose more vital fluid when it is already deficient.

We must keep in mind that our bodies have a very intelligent, well-designed, comprehensive system to maintain homeostasis under normal circumstances. If the body spontaneously begins to sweat excessively, one should consult a TCM doctor to check where there might be an imbalance. Or, if the body does not sweat enough due to weather changes, or due to "man-made weather" (such as air conditioning during the summer), then the body does not sweat enough to clean the skin and bring Qi circulation to the surface. Then it is good to promote perspiration in a natural way, such as with exercise or a hot bath or sauna.

6. The Lymphatic System

The lymphatic system is a filter and a defensive system. The lymph channels and nodes have many T- and B-cells, and other natural killer cells to destroy pathogens and abnormal and cancerous cells from both internal and external sources. The waste or toxins from the lymphatic system then flow either to the circulatory system of the blood via the kidneys, or to the skin, to be discharged from the body.

The Principle of Detoxification

Whatever we do to our bodies, whether detoxifying, supplementing, or implementing another program, we should not ignore one principle: *Follow the natural laws of our bodies.* Otherwise, we will only do the body harm, over both the short and long term. Additional rules follow this principle:

a) Enhance the body's own natural capacity to detoxify by choosing an appropriate lifestyle, rather than implementing a one-time detoxifying program. If the body is balanced and healthy, with the full capacity to self-regulate, one should not undertake extra measures to force the body in some way, interrupting the body's natural rhythm. Every person is born with the natural ability to overcome disease. The key to success is making changes in small steps, by correcting unhealthy lifestyles and behaviors.

b) Follow the laws of Mother Nature. Sometimes we do need to give our body extra help to detoxify when there are signs of the accumulating toxins in the body; but still, one must follow the body's natural laws. Mother Nature, not allopathic medicine, cures ills. The human body comes with marvelous

regenerative systems that have great powers to heal, recover, and revitalize themselves—without any outside help. Self-healing is a basic capacity of all living beings. The primary cause of ill health is living contrary to the requirements of Mother Nature. We must follow the natural laws of the body, rather than forcing and interrupting them with harsh methods. Humans require time to adjust to changes; natural health and fitness increase by making small improvements over time, ultimately achieving significant results. Health is a journey rather than a destination.
c) Any physical detoxification needs to cleanse toxins from the digestive system first. Fasting and colon cleanses are not required for detoxification. The body has detoxification systems that work best under conditions of regularity. Eat a healthy diet with adequate amounts of water and fiber, and your body will detoxify naturally.
d) Emotional detoxification must be a part of the detoxification process. (See below)

Natural Detoxification Methods

1. Sweating for detoxification: Sweating is a functional process of the skin to detoxify the body.
  a) Exercise to assist sweating: Exercise at least once a week is recommended to promote sweating. Simply walking can generate 3-5 times more heat in the body. Body heat can be increased 10-20 times with moderate to intensive exercise. To balance increased body heat, the skin's pores open, releasing sweat and toxins.
  b) Take a hot sauna, soak your feet in hot water, or the best method is to use herbal steam to assist the body in sweating out toxins from the skin.
  c) Drink a hot beverage or hot soup to assist the sweating

www.bodyw...
mystique.
.com

69

90
94
97

20

29

167 – water

ASIAN PICKLES

process, especially during the winter season or if too much cold and raw food has been consumed, causing cold stomach pain and cramps. This method will treat the cold pain and promote perspiration. Some suggestions are adding ginger to soup or porridge, or using white pepper in noodle soup, or, specifically for cold stomach pain or menstrual cramps, drinking hot tea with dark brown sugar and ginger. Summer is the season during which the body should sweat naturally to detoxify and lose weight. Summer sweating expels phlegm, naturally balancing the body after its accumulation of phlegm in the winter and springtime, when the body does not naturally sweat. Be advised not to use air conditioning excessively during the summer.

2. Promote urination for detoxification:
   a)   <u>Drink enough water daily</u>. We all know that the fundamental thing to do for urination is to drink enough fluids. But knowing how much is enough depends on each individual, since one's activity level, body mass, etc. are all different. Some suggest that one should drink at least 2,000 ml, or eight 8-oz glasses, of water daily. However, for someone with congestive heart failure or declining kidney or liver function, this "standard" amount of water intake will do a great deal of harm. The easy way to make adjustments to the amount of water one should drink is to observe one's urine color. In a well-hydrated individual, urine color should be slightly yellow or clear.

   Develop the habit of drinking water throughout the day. Make sure that water is easily accessible and conveniently within reach. Drink water every two hours; do not wait until you have the feeling of thirst, as that indicates that the body has already become dehydrated and is sending out the "thirsty" signal to the central nervous system. In the elderly, the sense of taste and thirst declines, so that it is even more important for this age group to consume water and other liquids regularly.

b) Eat fruits and vegetables that have diuretic properties. TCM classifies these kinds of fruits and vegetables in the "draining and clearing heat" category. Examples are watermelon (promotes urination, clears summer heat stroke, and supplements body fluid), grapes, and cherries. There are many vegetables with a diuretic function, such as winter melon, cucumbers, Napa cabbage, dandelions, and lettuce.

c) Acupuncture, massage, and a hot pad on the lower abdomen promote urination. If there is difficult urination, with signs of water retention, acupuncture can assist a great deal by enhancing body energy for discharging extra water. Applying a hot pad or massaging the lower abdomen also assist with urination.

d) Drink tea for promoting urination. Corn silk tea is not only excellent for promoting urination, but for preventing kidney and gallbladder stones and lowering blood pressure. *Plantago asiatica* (*che qian cao*), which grows in many regions, is a powerful diuretic and clears toxins. Green tea, also a good diuretic, detoxifies the body and cleanses and softens the blood vessels.

Fresh fruits, vegetables, and herbal tea are all alkaline, which neutralizes the acidity (toxins and wastes) that is produced constantly in our bodies. Therefore, they have more health advantages than just drinking water to detoxify the body.

Similarly, green tea and mung bean soup also promote detoxification far better than water, both containing substances that clear toxins and infections. Mung bean soup is used in China to clear summer heat and cleanse the body of pesticides absorbed from the environment.

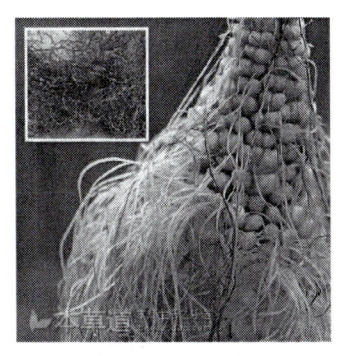

Corn silk (Zea mays l.)

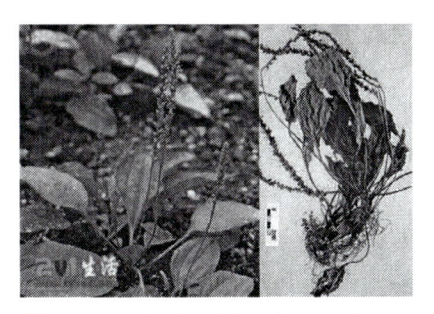

Plantago asiatica (che qian cao)

3. Promoting bowel regularity for detoxification:

a) Add more fiber to your diet. Before detoxifying the body or any specific organs, the most important first step is cleansing the digestive system, since it produces the most toxins. To detoxify naturally, increase consumption of filtered water, herbal teas, fruits, and vegetables and other fiber-rich foods, and reduce consumption of fats, red meats, and milk products. Adding fiber to your diet will help the body detoxify by promoting regularity. Eating fresh fruits and vegetables and high-fiber content foods, such as spinach, Napa cabbage, bamboo, cabbage, pumpkin, potatoes, and sweet potatoes, cleanses the bowels. The natural fiber from whole foods not only cleanses the gastroenterological system, but also absorbs and neutralizes toxins in the digestive system and provides nutrients to the body—something no artificial, "fiber-rich" commercial food can do.

b) A special food group: Seaweed, shiitake mushrooms, and black fungus mushrooms belong to a very special food group. They contain certain polysaccharides that stop the absorption of toxins into the body's digestive system, working like blood purifiers. Studies indicate that kelp and black fungus mushrooms can very effectively block the absorption of radioactive substances and contaminated food into the body.

They also promote bowel movements, reduce blood thickness, and soften the blood vessels. They are also rich in rare minerals. It is no wonder that this food group is one of the foods most commonly consumed by Chinese families.

4. Fasting for detoxification:

Fasting for detoxification has been practiced in many cultures for cleansing and detoxification purposes, and according to spiritual traditions. Fasting, or as the Chinese call it, *bi gu*, meaning "no grains," has been used for healing throughout the long history of China. It has been used as a healing method for cleansing the gastrointestinal system and detoxification, for expelling the extra, stagnant phlegm from the body, and to ensure and promote the free flow of Qi and blood after cleansing the phlegm. For this reason, since ancient times, the Chinese have practiced fasting to promote longevity. Fasting can also stimulate and revitalize the body's nervous and immune systems. Fasting for healing has to be practiced in a very gentle way, with the consumption of sufficient fluids, as well as some vegetables and fruits. The safest way is to find a reputable clinic or a specialist to instruct and supervise any fasting procedure.

Fasting contraindications for certain groups or conditions:
- a) Fasting is not recommended for children, the elderly, or pregnant and postpartum women.
- b) It is not advisable for people with certain medical conditions, such as cancer, particularly late-stage cancer; diabetes, in particular Type I diabetes with continued use of insulin; tuberculosis; severe liver, kidney, or heart disease, or hypertension due to kidney disease; severe ulcers in the digestive system; heart valve problems; those recovering from surgical procedures; those who are underweight or malnourished; or those who suffer mental disorders.

Gentle fasting can be done, such as eliminating dinner over the weekend, or eliminating one daytime meal 1-2 days per week. Whole-day fasting means not eating main foods like starch, proteins, and fats, but drinking sufficient liquids and eating some low-calorie fruits and vegetables, like cucumbers, apples, green leafy vegetables, turnips, celery, spinach, and carrots. Once the body is used to gentle fasting, one can gradually progress. There are many fasting schedules, gradually starting from easy to moderate, and not taking radical measures. During fasting, one should be stress-free, refrain from sexual activity, get sufficient liquids, and eat fruits and vegetables. After fasting, one should again gradually resume normal eating, first taking liquid food such as soup, then moving on to paste food, then to half the normal amount of solid food, then finally returning to your normal diet.

Fasting must be personalized, with a regimen based on each person's realistic goals and body condition. Otherwise, unsuitable fasting is nothing but another word for starvation. In starvation conditions, the body generates many wastes, metabolites, and toxins from the catabolization of proteins and fats. This can result in damage to the heart muscle and other organ tissues. The negative effects of fasting are greater in leaner than heavier individuals. In lean individuals, fasting results in a deterioration of glucose tolerance. The release of stored toxins in fatty tissues requires a fast of seven to ten days. Any fast lasting longer than three days should be supervised in a specialized inpatient facility.

5. Tea Drinking for Detoxification

There are thousands of kinds of teas from Mother Earth: green tea, white tea, black tea, and half-green/half-black (half-fermented) tea. Sometimes we use certain parts of herbs as herbal tea, or combine different herbs for therapeutic tea.

Benefits of drinking green tea:
   a) Green tea cleanses toxins, including radioactive toxins, by quickly discharging them from the body through the urine. In the laboratory, scientists have shown that green tea extract can inhibit certain bacteria, such as *Staphylococcus aureus*, *Vibrio cholerae*, and many *Enterobacteriaceae* that cause dysentery and gastroenteritis.
   b) Green tea maintains a healthy cardiovascular system. There are many active substances in tea that increase the elasticity of the blood vessels and help prevent heart disease by lowering triglycerides and cholesterol in the blood.
   c) Green tea helps prevent many cancers, including skin cancer. One should drink at least two cups of green tea per day to clean free radicals and other carcinogenic toxins from the body.
   d) Green tea is anti-aging. Green tea contains many rare minerals (selenium, silica, zinc, magnesium, potassium, sodium) and antioxidants, giving it detoxifying properties that help lower cholesterol and prevent heart disease (phlegm in the blood) and osteoporosis, thus slowing the aging process.

Note: One should drink freshly made tea, not tea left overnight. It is best to use whole, loose-leaf tea within one year of its harvest, rather than processed tea in a tea bag. Different teas need to be steeped at different temperatures. The finer and more tender the tea leaf, the lower the temperature of water used, in order not to destroy the many active substances in the tea. One can drink three times from the same tea leaf brew.

6. Vinegar for Detoxification

Chinese medicine uses rice vinegar for diet therapy, to prepare herbs for healing and disease prevention. A simple example is the use of vinegar in the vaporizer to prevent colds during the winter season.

Body without Mystique

Rice vinegar aids the digestive system to activate enzymes for digestion and assists the body to metabolize fatty foods for weight control. TCM doctors always advise patients, especially the elderly, to use more vinegar and less salt in their diet. Vinegar also assists skin circulation for beautiful skin, and inhibits the production of oxidization wastes, slowing down the aging process.

TCM doctors often use vinegar as a base mixed with herbs to make a paste to heal wounds and sports injuries.

How to use:
- Use rice vinegar, apple cider vinegar, or vinegar made from any grain (not synthetic); take 12-20 cc orally before and after breakfast. However, this is not recommended for people with acid reflux disease or a weak constitution.
- Mix vinegar with water and honey as a beverage.
- Use vinegar to soak certain foods for 10-30 days, and then eat the food.

Examples of vinegar in food therapy:
- **Peanuts and vinegar:** Soak raw peanuts in vinegar for one week, then eat 10 peanuts twice a day to lower cholesterol, soften the blood vessels, reduce hypertension, and prevent heart disease.

- **Kelp and vinegar:** Cut fresh, clean kelp into thin threads and soak in vinegar in the refrigerator for 10 days. Eat as a side dish to treat constipation and prevent osteoporosis.

- **Winter garlic and vinegar:** It is a very old Chinese tradition to soak fresh garlic in rice vinegar on a special winter day (December 8th on the lunar calendar). It is put into the refrigerator for about 10 days (for those living in a warmer winter region, like California). The garlic will turn a light jade color and is very tasty as an aid to digestion, detoxification of the body, and for killing parasites. (For some reason, if the garlic is soaked in vinegar during a different season, there is no beautiful jade color, and it is not as tasty as when it is soaked in the winter.) This fresh, garlic-tasting vinegar can be used for healing and to detoxify the body.

7. Herbal Baths (Yao Yu 药浴) for Detoxification

Herbal baths have a long history in Chinese medicine, dating back to 1300 BC. Many famous doctors in the history of the dynasties continued to develop them as treatments and detoxification for a variety of diseases, for prevention, to maintain well-being, and for longevity. Herbal baths are not only for the whole body, but for specific parts of the body. In fact, the Chinese word for "herbal bath" has a collective meaning that includes herbal baths for the whole body, herbal seat baths, herbal local soaks, herbal steams, and herbal washes for skin infections and injuries. Even simply a warm bubble bath is good for the body to detoxify via the skin.

Some aging scientists conducted research about twenty years ago indicating that warm baths before sleeping at night can promote longevity and slow down aging. The research showed that there is a tremendous amount of bacteria on the skin and hair that is cleansed with a warm bath. These bacteria produce a great deal of toxins on the skin, especially at nighttime when we go to sleep, when immunity is at its lowest. These toxins contribute to the body's aging. A warm herbal bath not only relaxes the body for better sleep, but also eliminates toxins, as well as having other therapeutic properties depending on the properties of the herbs used.

8. Exercise for Detoxification

Benefits of Exercise for Detoxification:
- Increases body temperature by boosting its metabolism. The

body will then increase perspiration, regulating body temperature and discharging toxins.
- Promotes intestinal peristalsis, which increases bowel movements to discharge wastes. Regular exercise assists and enhances the body's natural regularity, so that laxatives, which interrupt and sometimes damage the mucosal lining structure of the intestine, are unnecessary.
- Promotes urination by increasing blood circulation and kidney filtration, assisting body detoxification.
- Increases breathing for more O_2/CO_2 exchange, and more oxygen is carried by hemoglobin to the tissues and organs, increasing body immunity and detoxification.
- Increases systemic blood circulation and speeds up lymphatic system circulation by local muscle contraction. The lymphatic system discharges toxins by destroying internal and external pathogens and harmful substances via blood circulation and through the skin.

Exercises that Assist Body Detoxification:
- **Slow jogging and fast walking**
  This is the best way to burn more calories, promote sweating, and increase lymphatic circulation. It is best to exercise in nature with fresh air for lung detoxification and the beauty of the natural scenery for mental relaxation, rather than in the gym with recycled air and high noise levels. During fast walking, one can do deep, regular breathing and gentle coughing to clear the respiratory pathways, and move both arms to open up the chest.

  Note: If one expects to sweat a lot, drink water with a pinch of salt before starting your exercise. If there is a tendency to have muscle cramping, one can consume a calcium-rich beverage before exercising. After the exercise session, while the body is still sweating, do not take a cold shower right away, but rather, let the skin continue to sweat and cool down naturally before showering to prevent the stagnation of toxins in the body, pain in the muscles, fever, and even skin rashes. We all understand that after exercise, the body generates more heat, and the pores of the skin open to discharge toxins and heat. A sudden cold shower will stop this natural process, causing heat and toxins to stagnate under the skin, which can cause blockages and health problems.

- **Swimming and water aerobic exercises**
  Water reduces weight stress on joints by 90%. It is the best exercise for the elderly and for people with spinal cord and joint disorders. It is the best exercise for lung health and assists the lungs and the lymphatic system in detoxification.

  Note: It is best to wait for at least one hour after meals before swimming, and not to swim for over three hours at a time. During the summer, remember to protect the skin from the sun, and during the winter, it is best to swim in the early afternoon (during yang time), swimming slowly and with moderation.

- **Bicycling**
  This has the same benefit as fast walking and jogging by increasing blood circulation, sweating, and lymphatic circulation. Biking is a very good exercise, especially for people who have back or joint injuries.

- **Dancing and Tai Chi**
  These forms of exercise can be very enjoyable and mentally relaxing. It is good for stress reduction, balance, endurance, and increasing body/organ energy to assist in detoxification.

- **Other exercises**

    These can include taking every opportunity to walk up stairs rather than taking an elevator; jumping rope, for those who are very healthy; and stretching, particularly for people who work in front of a computer all day. It is beneficial to take five minutes to stretch every 1-2 hours.

    Note: These exercises are for assisting body detoxification, not for building muscle or heavy weight-lifting. The goal is good health, not competition or an aggressive workout that could stress or injure the body.

9. TCM Food Therapy for Detoxification

According to Chinese medicine, toxins come from the prolonged accumulation of phlegm, fire (heat or acidity), dampness, and mucus.

Types of Toxins: Substantial Toxins and Non-Substantial Toxins

Substantial toxins are those that can be seen visually, such as boils, pus, necrotic tissue, and discharge from the body. Non-substantial toxins consist mostly of the metabolites in our bodies, such as toxic chemicals, heavy metals, acids, uric acids, nitrates, aldehydes, ketones, and phenols.

Food that Detoxifies the Organs:

Food that cleanses the liver

The liver is the organ that filters and transforms toxins into less toxic or non-toxic substances in the body. However, if the liver is overworked or overloaded by toxins, or the liver function is compromised, such as by medication, a virus, or the prolonged use of alcohol, toxins will gradually accumulate in the body.

Maintaining healthy liver function and helping the liver to detoxify in a natural way should be practiced daily. There are many foods, such as carrots, garlic, grapes, figs, and corn silk tea that benefit the liver and help the liver to detoxify the body:

- **Carrots** help the liver detoxify mercury, lowering mercury levels in the blood and accelerating mercury discharge from the body. Beta-carotene, which the body converts into vitamin A, is especially important for eye health. It's also of great benefit to the skin, and the immune and digestive systems. Carrots are loaded with fiber and water, which cleanse the liver, boost detoxification, and plump out the skin to stave off wrinkles.

- **Garlic** detoxifies lead from the body.

- **Grapes** cleanse the liver and the digestive system.

- **Figs** benefit the liver by cleansing the digestion, aiding digestion, and helping the body to detoxify SO_2, SO_3, and other toxic chemicals from the body.

- **Corn silk tea** helps detoxify when there is an accumulation of toxins in the liver, and helps with cleansing jaundice and viral infections.

- Other beneficial foods for the liver include: bitter melon, mung beans, pumpkin, *Portulacae oleraceae* (*ma chi xian*), green tea, celery, and tomatoes.

Food that cleanses the kidneys:

The kidneys are very important organs in the body for discharging waste, especially metabolites from degraded proteins, and for maintaining homeostasis.

- **Cucumbers** help the kidneys clean toxic substances from the body, and clean the blood indirectly. Cucumbers also help the body clear the lungs, stomach, and liver organs. Cucumbers are a rich source of silica, a mineral needed for healthy skin, bone, and connective tissues. Silica also plays a major role in preventing cardiovascular disease and osteoporosis.

- **Cherries** help the kidneys clean and detoxify the body, and at the same time, help clean the bowels.

- **Red beans** are used in TCM for edema due to dampness and phlegm disease.

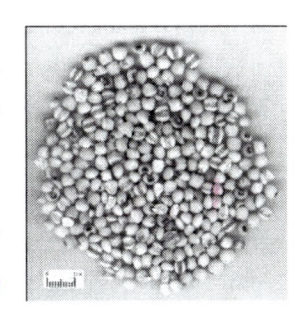

Pearl Barley

- **Pearl barley** helps treat edema.

- Other foods that benefit the kidneys include: black beans, watermelon, Napa cabbage, lily flowers, wild *Capsella bursa-pastoris* (shepherd's purse), grapes, white duck meat, and carp.

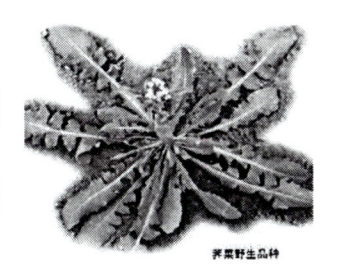

Shepherd's purse

<u>Food that cleanses the digestive system and helps with seafood poisoning:</u>

The GI system is the greatest toxin-producer in the body; the toxins then enter the blood via the portal vein system, and then directly enter the liver. This is why it is important to clean the GI tract before detoxifying any other organs, especially the liver.

When one has a regular bio-rhythm and a healthy diet, the body can keep its normal balance, without the accumulation of toxins in the body. If one eats an unhealthy diet, suffers from digestive system disorders, or abuses laxatives and frequently depends on colon therapies that interrupt the normal bio-rhythm of the digestive system, digestion and absorption function will decline, and more undigested food becomes available to the lower intestine, where more toxins will be produced.

TCM food therapy uses certain foods to help the digestive system detoxify and cleanse itself, such as black fungus mushrooms, the kelp family of sea vegetables, apples, strawberries, whole grains, and organic honey.

> **Black fungus mushrooms** (wood ear, cloud ear, and *Auricularia auricular-judae*) contain a lot of β-D polysaccharides. They can absorb toxins from the body via the GI tract and cleanse toxins from the body indirectly. One of the important functions of black fungus mushrooms is that they can slow down the body's absorption of and increase discharge of radioactive substances and contaminated food.
>
> **The kelp family of sea vegetables** includes some of the most consumed vegetables in Asia. They can halt GI tract absorption of the radioactive element silicon, preventing leukemia. They also absorb toxins in the body, helping it to detoxify.
>
> **Apples and strawberries** contain galactose aldehydic acids that detoxify the body and prevent production of toxins in the digestive system. Strawberries also have many kinds of fruit acids to cleanse the digestive system and assist the liver.
>
> **Honey** has been used in TCM for thousands of years to cleanse the GI tract, detoxify the body, and promote a beautiful facial complexion.
>
> **Other foods for cleansing the digestive system include:** Napa cabbage, spinach, bamboo, pumpkin, wild Chinese yams, and

potatoes.

Food that cleanses environmental toxins:
- Mung bean soup, fresh carrot juice, and green tea can clear pesticides absorbed into the body from the environment.
- Carrots have an active substance that can combine with mercury and discharge it from the body. They also help to lower cholesterol, maintain a healthy cardiovascular system, and increase body immunity.
- Chinese chives can clean silver poisoning.
- Water chestnuts soften and discharge copper.
- Kelp and black fungus mushrooms cleanse lead and radioactive poison from the digestive system.

Food that assists the body in defending against cancer:

Most foods that have the property of clearing heat and toxins have the greatest anti-cancer effects. These include mung beans, bitter melon, *ma chi xian* (*Portulaca*), pumpkin, kelp, black fungus mushrooms, garlic, onions, eggplants, turnips, and sweet potatoes (very good for longevity and anti-cancer). Other fruits and nuts that resist cancer growth include kiwis, figs, walnuts, citrus fruits, apricots, and hawthorn fruit.

Examples of food therapy for detoxification:

Detoxification Veggie Juice
Celery: 100g
Bitter melon: 50g
Carrots: 100g
One apple
Beets: 100g
Fresh ginger: 2 slices

Juice ingredients in a juicer. Drink daily for 10 days as one course of treatment. Repeat as needed.

Five-Flavored Soup
One piece of seaweed
Celery: 50g
One tomato
Water Chestnuts
Half an onion

Cut up all ingredients and add to water. Cook until soft. Add salt, fresh ginger, and spices as desired. Serve.

Seaweed Mung Bean Soup
Seaweed (kelp): 40g
Mung beans: 60g
Spices

Cook ingredients in water until the mung beans are soft and open. Serve.

Salad for Hypertension and Obesity
Fresh seaweed (kelp)
Celery 100g

Cut into pieces. Rinse with boiling water and drain. Add salt, sesame oil, fresh ginger, and any other spices you like. Serve.

Body without Mystique

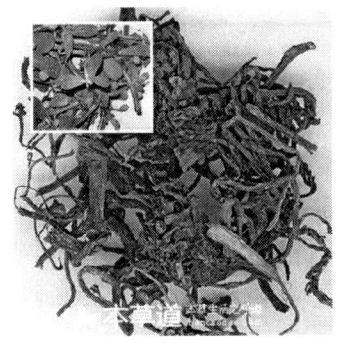

Ma chi qian (portulaca oleracea herba)

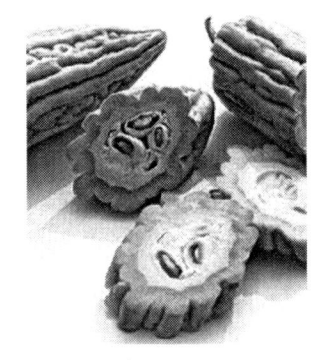

Bitter melon

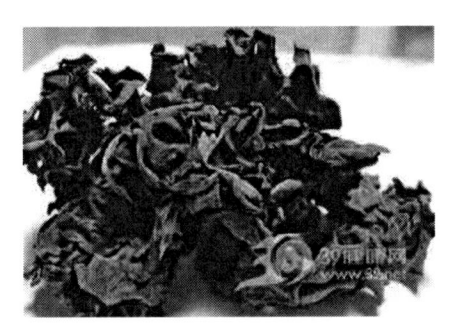

Black Fungus Mushrooms

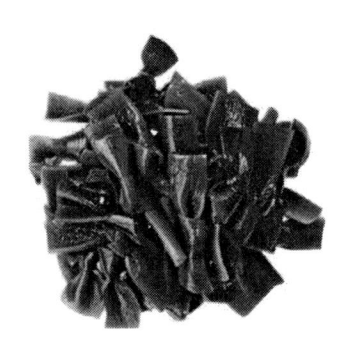

Kelp

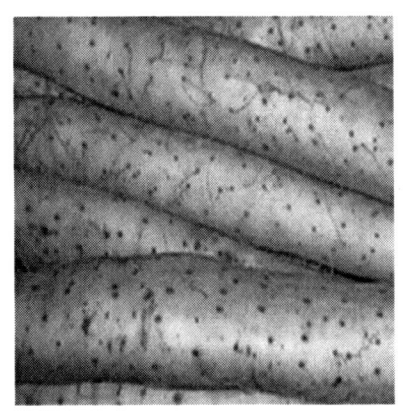

Shan yao (Chinese wild yam)

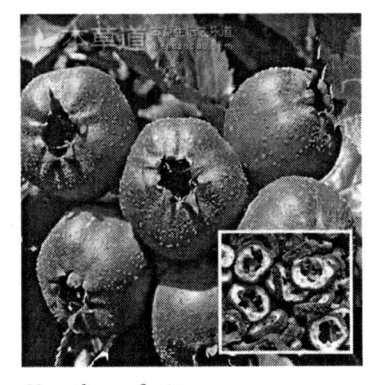

Hawthorn fruit

10. TCM Detoxification Therapies

<u>Massage for detoxification</u>

In general, massage therapy has been demonstrated to reduce anxiety, heart rate, and blood pressure. Massage also stimulates the immune system by increasing peripheral blood lymphocytes.

In China, massage has developed over the course of two thousand years to the present day. Chinese massage is called Tui Na Bone Setting Therapy. This massage is widely practiced and taught in hospitals and medical schools, both in TCM and in Western medical schools in China, where this osteopathic specialist training is an essential part of primary healthcare.

The TCM style of massage (Tui Na) is based on TCM meridian theory for specific health concerns. Tui Na therapy is a unique "longevity and well-being" specialty of TCM. It works on organ harmony, promotion of Qi and blood circulation, and increasing the body's immunity for longevity. It can be done by oneself or by a professional.

Here are some of the Tui Na methods that can be done by oneself:

- **Abdominal massage to promote bowel movements for detoxification**: Put your left hand over the back of your right hand and gently massage in a counter-clockwise direction 15-20 times, and then in a clockwise direction 15-20 times, and then from the upper abdominal area downward to the lower abdominal area 15-20 times. Finally, focus mentally on the umbilical area for 10 minutes.

    This abdominal massage works on the spleen, stomach, liver, and the Ren meridian. It increases Qi and blood circulation, harmonizes the organs, dissipates congestion and stasis in the organs, and assists bowel movement and detoxification.

    <u>Note</u>: Before performing abdominal massage, empty the

bladder. It also should not be performed if one is too hungry or has just eaten.

- **Kidney organ massage**: Warm up both your hands, then put them on each side of the lumbar area (lower back). Rub up and down from the lumbar to the tail bone 50-100 times, twice a day, in the morning and the night. Next, massage the bottoms of both feet until warm, then massage both ears until they are red and warm.

    These massages tonify kidney energy and warm the kidneys to assist the body in detoxification. They also assist in the treatment of menstrual disorders, premature ejaculation, and lumbar muscle and bone disorders.

- **Liver organ massage for detoxification**: Warm up both hands, then use three fingers to locate the hypochondriac area under the breast plate, along the top of the rib cage. Apply gentle pressure, pressing along the top of the rib cage. Both hands can cross over one another, or you can use the same hand to massage the hypochondriac area. Then massage both ring fingers at the third joint from the tip of the finger.

- **Foot Reflexology – hot herbal or hot water foot bath**: Reflexology is based on the principle that there are points in the hands and feet that correlate with organs, glands, and all the body systems. By stimulating these points, the body systems can be indirectly regulated. This is why it has been the custom in ancient China until the present day, as well as in many other cultures of the world, to soak and wash the feet in hot water. This is one of the best detoxification methods to balance and unblock distressed organs, as well as to promote circulation in the organs and assist draining the internal toxins from the body.

In the past, it was customary for Chinese families to use very hot water to soak the feet at night, the water being so hot that it made the person's face and forehead sweat. This ensured that the body's stomach meridian—from the feet, all the way up to the abdomen, chest, and face—would be totally opened up, promoting body detoxification. This detoxifying foot reflexology is a TCM therapy that works well for people who have insomnia, hypertension, or certain types of headaches due to toxic accumulation. Having detoxifying foot reflexology done regularly helps promote well-being and longevity.

Gua Sha Therapy

Gua Sha therapy is one of oldest folk therapies included in Traditional Chinese Medicine. A smooth-edged device—usually made from a water buffalo horn—is placed against the pre-oiled skin surface, pressed down firmly, and then moved down the muscles or along the pathway of the acupuncture meridians over the surface of the skin, until the skin reddens. The redness is called *Sha*; the darker the Sha, the more the blockage. The color of Sha varies according to the severity of the patient's blood stasis, which may correlate with the nature of energy stagnation inside the body, the severity, and the type of the disorder. The color can be a dark blue-black to a light pink, but is most often a shade of red. Although the marks on the skin look painful, they are not. Patients typically feel an immediate sense of relief from congestion and painful symptoms, such as influenza that causes head, neck, and shoulder pain with fever.

In classical Chinese practice, the Gua Sha technique is most commonly used to:
- Reduce fever (Gua Sha was used in China to treat cholera)
- Treat fatigue caused by exposure to heat (especially heat stroke) or cold
- Treat cough, dyspnea, bronchitis, asthma, and emphysema

- Treat muscle and tendon injuries
- Push sluggish circulation, or fibromyalgia
- Treat headaches
- Treat sunstroke/heat syncope and nausea
- Treat stiffness, pain, or immobility
- Treat digestive disorders
- Treat urinary and/or gynecological disorders
- Assist with reactions to food poisoning
- Assist in weight loss
- Rejuvenate facial skin

Note: Gua Sha therapy should avoid areas with big blood vessels, sense organs, the genital organs, and any wounds. After Gua Sha therapy, one should protect the treatment site and the neck from contact with the wind and cold.

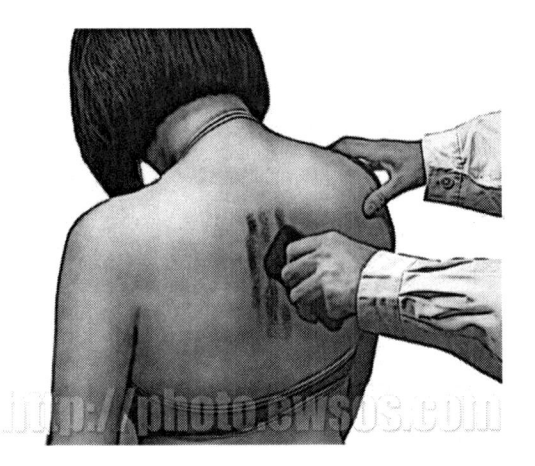

<u>Cupping</u>

Cupping is one of the oldest therapies practiced in many cultures, dating from as early as 3000 BC. It was described in 1550 BC by the Egyptians. In China, archaeologists have found evidence of cupping dating back to 1000 BC. In ancient Greece, circa 400 BC, cupping was used for internal diseases and structural problems. In multiple forms, this method spread into the medical practices of Asian and European civilizations.

Cupping locations and points are based on meridian theory and the injured location. If one of the organs is not functioning well and is imbalanced, there will be signs of deficiency or excess on the related meridian. Cupping treatment is then applied on the appropriate meridian to balance the internal organs. If there is blockage from stagnation in a certain area of the body, or an insect bite leaves toxic lesions on the skin, cupping can be a very effective treatment.

How cupping detoxifies the body: If an organ shows signs of stagnation and congestion, cupping can treat its related meridian, such as lung congestion during an infection, liver congestion from internal and external stressors, stress-related muscular channel/meridian blockages, and heat (toxin) accumulation. The cupping therapy will be applied along the congested meridian to decongest and unblock the organ-related pathway to restore free flow of Qi and blood, and balance the organs. Sometimes, people can see the benefit from the cupping therapy right away.

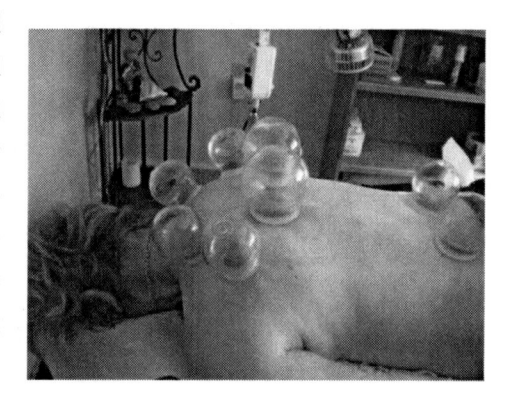

Note: There are some contraindications for cupping therapy, such as open wounds or proximity to large blood vessels, the five sense organs, or the genital area. After cupping therapy, one should protect the treatment site and the neck from contact with wind and cold.

Moxibustion

Moxibustion (*jiŭ*: 灸) is an important TCM therapy that uses moxa, or mugwort herb. It can be used indirectly, with acupuncture needles, or it is sometimes burned over the skin to warm a specific region or acupuncture point. It stimulates circulation through the points, inducing a smoother flow of blood and Qi. The free flow of Qi and blood can ensure that the body and organs function normally, are properly nourished, and discharge toxins and wastes. It is believed that moxibustion can stimulate blood flow in the pelvic area and uterus, and increases the body's immunity to assist it in detoxification. Moxibustion can work against cold and dampness in the body, treating many phlegm and cold-related health problems. Scientific research has shown that moxibustion:

1. **Increases the body's immunity.** Research studies with rabbits have shown increased activity of macrophage cells, increasing cell immunity by four times (4x) compared with the control group. Other research conducted on patients with chronic asthma showed that following moxibustion therapy, their T-cell proliferation rates increased from low levels back to normal.
2. **Treats allergies and autoimmune disorders.** Modern science still cannot explain why moxibustion treatment helps autoimmune disorders, but laboratory research has observed that the death rate in mice with autoimmune disorders goes from 90% to 10% with moxibustion treatment. Treatment reduces the number of mast cells and their vasoactive and inflammatory mediators.
3. **Helps the body fight cancer cells.** Moxibustion therapy can increase cell immunity, which is the principle means to fight cancer cells. Most cancer patients experience fatigue and nausea after chemotherapy; moxibustion can quickly restore the body's energy and soothe the stomach in the short term. In the longer term, moxibustion therapy restores immunity, increases blood count to prevent anemia, and prevents and/or reduces hair loss.
4. **Helps control bacterial infection.**
5. **Regulates the cardio-cerebral vascular system.** Moxibustion balances blood pressure. When a person is in a state of shock, with lowered blood pressure, moxibustion therapy on certain acu-points raises blood pressure back to normal levels. Contrarily, it can also lower blood pressure from high to normal levels. Moxibustion relaxes the blood vessels and changes blood flow and force, benefitting circulation in the heart and the brain.
6. **Regulates the hematological system.** Research undertaken in

Japan indicates that white blood cell count increases 2-3 times more than normal 1-4 hours after moxibustion therapy. It also shows increased red blood cell count and hemoglobin count up to one week after therapy, with continued significant increases for an average of eight weeks following treatment.
7. **Helps control pain**.
8. **Helps women with premenstrual syndrome** (PMS) and other chronic health problems, such as infertility, fetal malposition in expectant mothers, and perimenopausal and menopausal problems.

Herbal Baths (see description on page 98)

11. Taking Supplements for Detoxification

The body already naturally has a sophisticated system for self-detoxification, so what we call "supplement" means supplying something to the body that it is incapable of producing for itself, or that it somehow lacks. Since the body has its own system, or energy, for detoxification, if we have a healthy lifestyle and well-balanced nutrition, it has everything it needs to take care itself. However, if we are to take supplements to assist the body in detoxification, the following are some suggestions I would like to give my readers:

1) If a supplement is made from regular fruits, vegetables, or some other edible plant, it is best to eat the whole, fresh fruit or vegetable. For example, it is much better to eat fresh blueberries and dark grapes, rather than paying hundreds of dollars for bottled supplements, which often contain preservatives.

   For example, taking fish oil capsules is unnecessary if one eats fresh salmon once or twice a week. Add spices such as garlic to your normal cooking, rather than taking capsules of processed garlic that have far less nutrition than fresh, or even cooked, garlic. Make fresh celery and beet juice before taking blood pressure pills when exhibiting the early stages of hypertension—and celery capsules definitely won't do. Drink one or two cups of green tea to detoxify the body, soften the blood vessels, help lose weight, lower cholesterol, and protect the skin from environmental toxins. Again, green tea capsules cannot compare with the medicinal properties of fresh green tea.

Research indicates that natural, unprocessed herbs have 100% efficacy, whereas, after being processed and made into supplements, they retain only 50% efficacy. Even using a sophisticated process and a relatively low temperature to process these products, there is still a reduction of 20-25% efficacy. Such processing also adds significantly to the final cost of the completed products.

We should understand that the healthiest, simplest, and most economical approach is to consume balanced, whole, fresh foods that provide most of the elements we need.

2) Do intensive research to find out what the normal dosage is for different age groups and to find out what the side effects may be if one takes too much of a particular supplement.

As an example: After seeing a variety of healthcare practitioners in some well-known institutes, Mary came to the office for a consultation. She had been feeling chronically fatigued and stressed and had some body pain. Mary did not want to take any prescription medication, so her doctor sold her a lot of supplements. One supplement for fatigue had a high dosage of vitamins, from A-Z; the next supplement was for muscle pain, or possibly fibromyalgia, again with a high dosage of vitamins; the last supplement was for PMS, again with a high dosage of vitamins. After adding all the vitamins together, Mary had been taking somewhere between 3,000-

5,000% more than a normal adult should take! This is not to mention the binding substances in the vitamins. Our organs—the digestive system, liver, and kidneys—have to work extra hard in order to expel excess. After she had stopped taking any of her supplements for a week, Mary felt a lot more energetic, with less pain in her body.

3) Find out if the supplement contents are contraindicated to any of the medications you may currently be taking.

4) Ask yourself if you really need the supplement, or if, for whatever reason, someone is making a sell—be they your doctor, alternative medicine practitioner, chiropractor, yoga teacher, or a multi-level marketing group.

    <u>Always remember: No matter how good a supplement may be, if it is not suited for your body and your specific needs, you are not only wasting money, but burdening your body without benefit.</u>

5) If you are taking a supplement for a certain purpose, make sure to discontinue it after your health concern is resolved, or be sure to stop taking it if you do not see any benefit after having taken it for a while.

6) If you do take a supplement or supplements over a long period of time, consider the following:

    - The best way is to take the supplements for several months, then stop for a few months before resuming them again.
    - The winter season is the best season for taking supplements. During the winter, the body's energy goes inward, so it is the best time to replenish the body's reserves.

However, during the summer, our digestive system is relatively weaker, so too much supplement usage will reduce the appetite and further weaken digestion.

- Whenever you catch cold or have digestive problems or other health issues, first stop your supplements and then consult your healthcare practitioner to deal with the health issue. After the acute stage of the sickness has passed, you can then resume taking your supplements.

What is the difference between a Chinese herbal formula and other herbal supplements?

A Chinese herbal formula is a unique combination of herbs, based upon Chinese medical theory and the pattern diagnosis of organ disharmony for an individual made by a TCM doctor. An experienced TCM doctor must first evaluate the patient to make a pattern diagnosis and then formulate a prescription by selecting a combination of herbs that work together synergistically. The classic herbal formula is composed of a unique system of first selecting the "chief herb" that targets the most prominent problem of the affected organ, then selecting the "deputy herbs" to assist the chief herb in conducting its main task and to take care of and treat the comparatively minor problems associated with the main disharmony. Then the "assistant herbs" are assigned to balance out the harshness and potential side effects of the chief and deputy herbs. Finally, the "conveying herbs" are used to internally harmonize the herbal formula as a whole and convey them to the targeted organ. Once the body gets well from taking the herbal formula, one should stop taking it.

Taking herbal supplements, on the other hand, is an entirely different concept, similar to the belief that one should supplement with vitamins to avoid deficiencies of certain nutrients in the body. First of all, herbal supplements that are purchased over-the-counter contain only one or two herbs that may perform certain tasks and treat symptoms, but they will not address the cause of the health problem. This is why many people do not get any benefit by way of herbal supplementation; rather, the cause of the health problem or symptoms must be properly ascertained and treated.

In fact, the taking of supplements overall follows the same principle found in Western medicine, the idea of a "magic bullet" that works for everyone. With this "one size fits all" mentality, everyone gets the same supplement for the same symptoms, regardless of the underlying cause of the problem or one's body constitution, age, or gender.

12. Psychological/Emotional Detoxification

Inner Classic explains that spiritual (sheng) activity manifests a state of well-being and balances the body and the organs. In other words, spiritual life can greatly influence the state of the body and the organs. It has been believed and taught throughout all of TCM history that one of the most important principles for promoting longevity and well-being and to prevent disease is to have a strong spiritual will and purpose. In this way, one develops a good spirit, integrates body and soul, adapts more readily to the environment and to heat and cold, and harmonizes joy and anger (the emotions).

As we can see and experience in our modern society, we can bring about many disastrous effects to our physical, psychological, spiritual, financial, and environmental relationships from wanting ever more: from being greedy, wanting more power, having more desires and expectations, feeding self-righteousness and ego, and so on, without end.

There are many paths (Dao: 道) to balance the emotions, to detoxify negative mental activity, and to enrich your spiritual life. These may be through spiritual practice, meditation, Tai Chi, yoga, prayer, or otherwise building a strong faith. One can continue to study and search for meaning and purpose for the development of inner peace, happiness, and personal well-being.

Stressful environments (including internal, external, physical, and psychological environments), whether short- or long-term, cause more than 60% of the health problems found in our modern society. Spiritual practice and meditation can be part of stress and anxiety reduction.

One of the characteristics of our busy modern lives is that we become more individualistic and isolated, and have weaker bonds with family, relatives, and friends. A common option is to seek help from a professional psychologist in order to empower oneself for healing and for help in building stronger relationships with family and relatives, as well as stronger friendships that provide positive psychological and emotional support. Participation in community activities, helping others, and supporting a good cause, such as working for a better earth and peace in the world, can have many positive rewards. In the process of lifting the spirit and finding inner peace and a joyful attitude in giving back to humanity, we can avoid and eliminate negativities of many kinds.

Natural health and wellness is a way of life available to everyone. It is about promoting personal health and fitness through the natural therapies of a healthy diet, appropriate nutritional supplementation, beneficial exercise, and a healthy attitude and positive spiritual life. Healthy living and patience promote personal health and fitness.

CPSIA information can be obtained at www.ICGtesting.com
Printed in the USA
BVOW021417030613

322309BV00019B/576/P